MANAGING DIABETES

BIOPOLITICS: MEDICINE, TECHNOSCIENCE, AND HEALTH IN THE TWENTY-FIRST CENTURY SERIES

General Editors: Monica J. Casper and Lisa Jean Moore

Missing Bodies: The Politics of Visibility
Monica J. Casper and Lisa Jean Moore

Against Health: How Health Became the New Morality
Edited by Jonathan M. Metzl and Anna Kirkland

Is Breast Best? Taking on the Breastfeeding Experts and the New High Stakes of Motherhood
Joan B. Wolf

Biopolitics: An Advanced Introduction
Thomas Lemke

The Material Gene: Gender, Race, and Heredity after the Human Genome Project
Kelly E. Happe

Cloning Wild Life: Zoos, Captivity, and the Future of Endangered Animals
Carrie Friese

Eating Drugs: Psychopharmaceutical Pluralism in India
Stefan Ecks

Phantom Limb: Amputation, Embodiment, and Prosthetic Technology
Cassandra S. Crawford

Heart-Sick: The Politics of Risk, Inequality, and Heart Disease
Janet K. Shim

Plucked: A History of Hair Removal
Rebecca M. Herzig

Contesting Intersex: The Dubious Diagnosis
Georgiann Davis

Men at Risk: Masculinity, Heterosexuality, and HIV Prevention
Shari L. Dworkin

To Fix or To Heal: Patient Care, Public Health, and the Limits of Biomedicine
Edited by Joseph E. Davis and Ana Marta González

Mattering: Feminism, Science, and Materialism
Edited by Victoria Pitts-Taylor

Are Racists Crazy? How Prejudice, Racism, and Antisemitism Became Markers of Insanity
Sander L. Gilman and James M. Thomas

Contraceptive Risk: The FDA, Depo-Provera, and the Politics of Experimental Medicine
William Green

Personalized Medicine: Empowered Patients in the 21st Century
Barbara Prainsack

Biocitizenship: On Bodies, Belonging, and the Politics of Life
Edited by Kelly E. Happe, Jenell Johnson, and Marina Levina

Toxic Shock: A Social History
Sharra L. Vostral

Managing Diabetes: The Cultural Politics of Disease
Jeffrey A. Bennett

Managing Diabetes

The Cultural Politics of Disease

Jeffrey A. Bennett

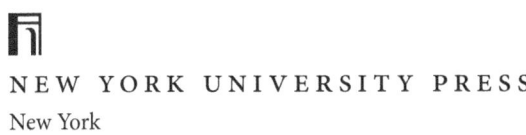
NEW YORK UNIVERSITY PRESS
New York

NEW YORK UNIVERSITY PRESS
New York
www.nyupress.org

© 2019 by New York University
All rights reserved

References to Internet websites (URLs) were accurate at the time of writing. Neither the author nor New York University Press is responsible for URLs that may have expired or changed since the manuscript was prepared.

Library of Congress Cataloging-in-Publication Data
Names: Bennett, Jeffrey A. (Jeffrey Allen), 1974– author.
Title: Managing diabetes : the cultural politics of disease / Jeffrey A. Bennett.
Description: New York : New York University Press, [2019] | Includes bibliographical references and index.
Identifiers: LCCN 2018041801| ISBN 9781479830435 (cl : alk. paper) | ISBN 9781479835287 (pb : alk. paper)
Subjects: LCSH: Diabetes—Treatment.
Classification: LCC RC660 .B386 2019 | DDC 616.4/62—dc23
LC record available at https://lccn.loc.gov/2018041801

New York University Press books are printed on acid-free paper, and their binding materials are chosen for strength and durability. We strive to use environmentally responsible suppliers and materials to the greatest extent possible in publishing our books.

Manufactured in the United States of America

10 9 8 7 6 5 4 3 2 1

Also available as an ebook

For Isaac,
who keeps life sweet

CONTENTS

1. Critical Conditions	1
2. "HIV Is the New Diabetes": Analogies of Apathy	42
3. Lethal Premonitions: Fatalism and Advocacy	77
4. Containing Sotomayor: Narratives of Personal Restraint	112
5. Troubled Interventions: "Epidemic" Logic and Institutional Oversight	142
6. Cyborg Dreams	173
Acknowledgments	203
Notes	207
Index	239
About the Author	247

1

Critical Conditions

Besides, I think that the cicadas, who are singing and carrying on conversations with one another in the heat of the day above our heads, are also watching us. And if they saw the two of us avoiding conversation at midday like most people, diverted by their song and, sluggish of mind, nodding off, they would have every right to laugh at us, convinced that a pair of slaves had come to their resting place to sleep like sheep gathering around the spring in the afternoon. But if they see us in conversation, steadfastly navigating around them as if they were Sirens, they will be very pleased and immediately give us the gift from the gods they are able to give to mortals.
—Socrates, Plato's *Phaedrus*, 259A–259E

As soon as you awake, the familiar pressure is there: Should you write or not? Yes, no, maybe. You heave your body out of bed, prick your finger, and squeeze a drop of blood onto the glucose meter. You shoot insulin into your stomach, eat, go for a walk. You concentrate on your feet touching the ground, on the blue stretch of sky, the roar of crashing waves, the pungent odor of guano. You listen to the environment as Don Juan urged Castaneda to do. Searching for analogies to your budding ideas, you scan cypress trees with twisted trunks, a flock of pelicans flying low over the water, breakers shooting up the cliff walls like geysers.
—Gloria Anzaldúa, *Light in the Dark/Luz en lo Oscuro*

The song of the cicadas murmured through the streets of Bloomington, Indiana in the summer of 2004. After 17 years hibernating underground, the creatures extolled in Plato's ode to rhetoric, madness, and love trumpeted their return with harmonious fervor. I vividly remember walking past the trees that lined the path from Ballantine Hall to the parking lot behind the Kinsey Institute, distracted by their rapturous hymn. The cicadas' ubiquitous and ethereal orchestration crescendoed from a subtle whisper to an intense reverberation in a matter of steps. They animated the branches by giving them a pulse, enlivening the atmosphere with an energy that was somehow both electrifying and soothing. The hum from the trees was nothing short of overwhelming, imparting the feeling that at any moment they might conspire to overtake the walkway and whoever happened to be occupying it. Though invisible, they loomed large, effortlessly altering the scene with their euphoric chorus.

In ancient Greece cicadas represented spiritual ecstasy, rebirth, and immortality. Plato invokes the image of the cicadas in the *Phaedrus* to symbolize both restraint and honor, narratively crafting a link between personal control and dignity. Plato's protagonist Socrates tells his companion, the book's namesake Phaedrus, that they must resist the song of the cicadas, not succumbing to laziness, but practicing restraint against the pleasure-inducing cadence of the insects. Those familiar with the text know that Socrates is obsessing over his libido more than he is lauding some bugs in a plane tree. The storied philosopher reels in his desires for the titillating youthfulness of Phaedrus as he advocates for a disciplining of the passions and the virtue to be cultivated as a result. Socrates hopes that the cicadas will relay to the Muses his moderation and chaste disposition, and that he will be rewarded by Erato, the muse of love, and Calliope, the muse of rhetorical eloquence. Desires constantly encroach on Socrates, and he reproaches these temptations with overt gestures of self-control.

The relationship between duty and pleasure, what scholars frequently denote as hedonics, is a recurring theme in this book, which is dedicated to the manifestation and circulation of diabetes rhetoric. The tension between earthly desire and the platitudes of well-being is one I learned firsthand when I was diagnosed with type 1 diabetes the same summer the cicadas were resurrected in southern Indiana. Just a few weeks after defending my dissertation (a study about the relationship between blood and politics no less), the droning from the cicadas continued to stir as I was hospitalized suddenly after lower-back pain left me unable to sit, stand, or lay down comfortably. The pain was unlike anything I had experienced up to that point in my life and it still haunts me when I have the slightest backache. Because I was unaware that I had onset diabetes, my blood sugar was unregulated, inciting a condition known as ketoacidosis. In short, my kidneys had begun shutting down. I was immediately admitted to the ICU and spent a dizzying 48 hours immersing myself in a new language, a new routine, and a new way of life.

There were plenty of signs that trouble was on the horizon in the weeks leading up to my hospitalization, but they were not yet intelligible as something that might signify disease, illness, or however we want to classify diabetes in the medical order of things.[1] For starters, I suffered perpetual exhaustion. Having just finished a dissertation, landed a job, and started the emotionally taxing task of finding a new home in a distant city while saying good-bye to my grad school kin, including my partner of just over a year at the time, I wrote off the fatigue as a by-product of stress. I was also terribly moody. Although I am a reliably easygoing person, I found myself regularly irritated. The hormonal changes that accompanied diabetes's awakening left me undone, conjuring emotions that generally remained dormant in otherwise mundane situations. I had also lost a good bit of weight, but I tended to exercise frequently and was conscious of the scale, so again I attributed the weight loss to stress. When the doctors told me that I weighed a mere 120 pounds as a 5-foot,10-inch-tall man approaching age thirty, I was taken aback. The Greek word for diabetes translates to "siphon," and the disease was living up to its etymological signifier.

The weeks and months that followed diagnosis were accompanied by a steep learning curve about diabetes care, but also a newly found appreciation for gauging my body's response to fluctuating circumstances. Like all people with diabetes, I learned how to count carbohydrates, test my blood sugar, and administer shots. The finger pricks and shots were especially confounding, as I had lived for years with a pronounced phobia of needles. So strong was this aversion that I refused local anesthetics at the dentist's office before having my teeth drilled for fillings. One of the nurses working with me early in my diagnosis quipped, "A diabetic who doesn't like needles—how's that working out for you?" Of all the medical conditions that I could have landed, this one seemed decidedly cruel, as if I was the butt of some cosmic joke. Clearly, the cicadas had delivered bad news to the wrong muse.

There were other complications that I could not foresee. Early on, my pancreas was still producing trace amounts of insulin (a normal phenomenon for those with type 1 diabetes) and when it interacted with the insulin I was manually injecting, it caused me to have unusual balance problems. I remember on one job interview shortly after diagnosis having a difficult time focusing on a senior scholar's face as she posed a question. Although I was supposed to be answering her inquiries thoughtfully, I recall struggling to maintain composure and not embarrass myself during a dizzy spell. Driving and public speaking both became precarious endeavors because any mild change in heart rate or nerves left me unsure of whether my sugars were spiking or dropping rapidly. A friend from graduate school warned my partner to monitor me for depression, knowing that the first year after being diagnosed with a disease, chronic or otherwise, can leave a person despondent. I never pursued treatment or clarity about depression, worrying that any trace of flexibility in my concept of self would suggest that I was unable to contend with the multitude of changes I was juggling. Still, that first year I slept more than was normal, I lost time in ways I never had, and I became preoccupied with the life-altering ailments that awaited me. Assurances that "there are worse diseases you could have" or "things aren't like they used to be" only made matters worse. In the years prior to the Affordable Care Act, I also worried that formal recognition of depression might be used against me in future health insurance matters. I grappled with the fallout of the diagnosis for years, consuming as much information as I could about cures (and some scientist is always curing some poor mouse of something), technological innovations, and the prospects of a long and healthy life.

But what caught me most off guard in those first months were the disturbing ways people in every realm of my life, from close friends to complete strangers, communicated about diabetes. Even the most well-intentioned conversations about diabetes quickly devolved into recitations about the need to "take care" of myself, a variation of a conventional narrative about personal responsibility and hard work. The number of people who told me stories about relatives who *had* diabetes, always in the past tense, was legion. On airplanes, in restaurants, during office hours, and at the gym (!) people implored me to be attentive to my body. Although I rarely engaged with those who attempted to discipline what I ate, what some people with diabetes call "hand slapping," I commonly heard about death, folks who went blind from sugar irregularities, and the trope of the irresponsible diabetic who threw to the wind any thought of deliberate management. Sometimes the subjects of these cautionary tales were older men who had lost a foot to diabetes. At other times they were teenagers who died while in high school. One well-meaning relative told me the story of an acquaintance who had gone blind before dying from diabetes-related complications. Noticing the look of dismay on my face, she quickly added, "He was a crack addict too, though." Of course, these stories of loss are generally heart-wrenching for the people sharing them. They disclose their experiences in the hopes that my loved ones and me might avoid the pain they endured and the misfortunes they witnessed. Still, it is little wonder that depression hits hard in the first year after diagnosis. On the one hand, people with diabetes are told their disease is not so bad; on the other hand, it is conveyed repeatedly as fatal. Deciphering which messages are pertinent to the immediacy of one's livelihood can be a daunting undertaking when attempting to stay well.

Along with these dispiriting exchanges I was fast learning that vigilance did not always produce the results that I presumed and most certainly did not ensure the consistency narrativized about diabetes by others. I'm about as predictable as a human being can be. And yet, repetitive practices did not engender the effects typically described in medical literature. Early in my diagnosis I discovered that the same routine could produce glucose readings that were 100–150 points apart.[2] I found that diabetes management is not merely about counting carbohydrates and administering insulin but is complicated by factors such as a lack of sleep, stress, exercise, caffeine, and a host of idiosyncratic circumstances. As Annemarie Mol notes, in the logic of diabetes care, "no variable is ever fixed."[3] People with diabetes can mind these variations, but the plasticity of the disease is readily glossed over by those who have rigid predispositions about its effects. Even worse, these personal complexities can be dismissed as merely anecdotal.[4]

The inconsistent outcomes that emerged from my daily activities stood in sharp contrast to the facts I was cultivating about diabetes. Methodical patterns were supposed to produce steady results. When that did not happen, I found myself internalizing feelings of shame for not having an appropriate amount of self-control. But, even more significant, I realized that while I was suffering a degree of mortification about my increasingly unchecked numbers, I also had the sneaking suspicion that this narrative about a lack of personal restraint would inevitably be used to blame me for my own demise. I mean, how many of you have attended a funeral where someone uttered the words, "he just didn't take care of himself." I've been to more than a few. Couple that with the fact that I have never been averse to sin and the recipe for scapegoating was ripe. I could just picture the bereaved whispering at my wake, "You know how much fast food he ate, don't you?" "If Facebook is any indication, he always seemed to be drinking with friends." "He was diagnosed the day after eating at a Cheesecake Factory, what does that tell you?" It is the casualness of dismissal that haunts me most when thinking about diabetes rhetoric, the assumption that the care of the self is easily executed, even as nuanced understandings about the contours of "management" are elided. This paradigm is at best wickedly deceptive and at worst callously malicious—just "take care of yourself" and everything else will fall into place. I find this discourse resoundingly dubious because lurking just below the surface is an acknowledgment that control is achievable only after bracketing some of the most byzantine factors related to healthy living—the sociality of eating, the high cost of fresh food, the dark side of well-being regimens, and the mammoth and impenetrable nature of the healthcare system.[5] The almost compulsive urge to guide people's behavior reveals that the constructed nature of "health" can be just as diabolical as any disease.[6]

And I've got type 1 diabetes—the kind that supposedly lives free of blame because it is technically an autoimmune disease and not attributed to diet or "lifestyle" choices. People with type 2 diabetes are damned constantly by moralizers who insist their condition is one of their own making. It is regularly assumed that people with type 2 diabetes ate too much, exercised too little, and ultimately initiated their own downfall. Although this is sometimes true, it is an oversimplification of a dynamic chronic condition that is best addressed free of persecutory accusations. Even among some type 1 communities there is a desire to rename one of the two diseases and do away with the guilt by association that accompanies such noxious public judgments. If only the language that constitutes diabetes could be made more transparent, the thinking goes, then certainly we could escape disparaging glares and indelicate remarks, not to mention make medical strides to cure both diseases.

This book argues against such thinking, contending that the symbol system guiding diabetes rhetoric is, to borrow a phrase from Paula Treichler, marked by a crisis of signification.[7] Disparate visions of diabetes and its management circulate unceasingly and inharmoniously in public culture, contributing to a confusion, if not opaque mystification, about the disease. Depending on the source, diabetes might be imagined as an "epidemic" that necessitates government interference and multilevel task forces. For others, it is not so much a biopolitical question of state regulation, but the failure of individuals to exercise self-discipline. In some outlets, diabetes is positioned as thoughtlessly managed by swallowing a pill or programming a pump. In still other locations the disease is conceived as a dire state-of-being, a slow death that imperceptibly foments bodily decay. Diabetes is a banal and gradual disease, but couched recurrently in metaphors stressing war, natural disaster, addiction, and criminality. It is sometimes heralded as a product of nature, sometimes nurture, and sometimes both. In the medical literature, diabetes's catalyst is itself unknown, attributed to everything from viruses to gut bacteria to hormones to environmental toxins to some combination thereof.[8] Healthcare workers extol the promise of new innovations, such as insulin pumps, but also expend much energy worrying that people will attach such devices without reflection and abandon their duties of self-care. These contradictions occlude the fact that the paths to making a better life with diabetes are as diverse as the people who live with it.

This text does not strive to solve the inherent contradictions that organize diabetes's strange public life. Rather, I look to the trope of *management* as an instance of condensation, in the rhetorical sense, that helps to smooth over the discrepancies that mark the ways diabetes is made intelligible.[9] Put another way, management operates as a shorthand for multiple rhetorics that deal with sociality, relationality, food consumption, institutional support, ideologies of health, medical directives, and, perhaps most important, moral worth. Entering the labyrinth of diabetes management reveals its contours to be more serpentine than transparent, riddled with discrepant messages and incommensurable impulses. Giving attention to diabetes's puzzling incoherencies can trouble visions of self-sovereign subjects endowed with limitless personal agency and elucidate the cultural forces that help to structure life with the disease. Messages about diabetes circulate promiscuously and materialize in ways that are sometimes empowering, frequently disconcerting, and habitually more convoluted than envisioned in everyday exchanges and media representations. The forces shaping diabetes are polyvalent, customarily progressive and conservative simultaneously, sanctioning and restricting cultural inclinations about its enigmatic contours.[10]

Managing Diabetes attends to commonplace figurations of management to discern how routine meaning-making practices enliven the possibilities for judgment about diabetes outside a narrowly conceived medical model. Focusing on clinical presumptions of diabetes tends to reproduce rote notions of restraint, discipline, and mortification. However, such an emphasis does little to address equally significant incarnations of the disease or help us to understand why public misperceptions of diabetes continue unabated. Using a series of case studies, I look beyond the clinic to engage how management paradigms disseminate among publics and, in the process, reinforce some interpretations of the condition while disregarding others. Scrutinizing management's parameters can both disrupt taken-for-granted notions about the ease of control and better equip people with diabetes to navigate how their bodies are surveilled by those promoting well-being regimens. The rhetorical architecture of management helps to explain why some policies are privileged over others, why some forms of activism are effective and others are not, and why some technologies are adopted as curative while others are rendered obsolete. Diabetes's formidable presence is sustained by a host of social, cultural, and economic articulations. And that complex array of significations, brought to life by the composite structure of "management," is where we begin.

Diabetes: A Crisis of Signification

Humanistic, social scientific, and medical investigations of health teach us that the ways we communicate about disease and illness have a direct effect on how we act upon them. When I submit that management is a condensation of disparate referents, I simply mean that diabetes can only be known through a language that is stretched to generalize across millions of bodies. The constitutive power of language to formulate attitudes and conceptualize strategies for care is not merely descriptive, but essential to diabetes's mystifying qualities. Narratives, anecdotes, and myths are decisive in their ability to energize patient feelings, guide medical deliberations, and arrange classificatory hierarchies. Consider the following pieces of information, each of which actualizes diabetes in specific ways, but which are also collectively greater than the sum of their parts: More than 29 million people in the United States, in excess of 9 percent of the population, have some form of diabetes.[11] That's more than the number of people who live in the state of Texas. Of that, more than 8 million people remain undiagnosed, which is roughly the equivalent of Virginia's population. Adults with diabetes are two to four times more likely to die of heart disease or have a stroke than those without it. As a result, life expectancy rates are seven to ten years shorter for people with the condition. Diabetes is the leading cause of blindness and kidney failure for adults and is the source of roughly two-thirds of all nontraumatic lower-limb amputations. People with diabetes are also twice as likely to experience depression as those without it.[12] Minority communities and economically marginalized populations continue to be ravaged by the disease and its devastating consequences in disproportionate numbers. Diabetes costs the United States about $327 billion annually in lost wages, healthcare expenditures, and related factors.[13]

These statistics delineate one way that diabetes can be made intelligible, feeding narratives with expectations, urgency, and obstacles that narrow the focus of its symbolic and material parameters. What is more unclear but equally significant is the effect this cumulative data has on public perceptions of the condition. The above statistics outline trauma and despair, lending an air of inevitability about the chances of survival. What are we to believe about the livelihood of those with diabetes if the above figures are privileged? Might these measures affect their everyday habits? Could this avalanche of information contribute to feelings of embarrassment, rates of depression, and resistance to medical advice? In isolation from other considerations these figures could denote a structural rendition of disease that relies on the biopolitical power of statistics to chart patient compliance and health outcomes. The numbers most certainly frame diabetes as a national crisis, influencing allegories about the purity of the homeland, the alleged dissolution of the nation's work ethic, and even the perceived standing of the United States as a global superpower.[14] The gravity of public narratives is puissant and the above statistics become meaningful when articulated to socially sanctioned truths: that control can always be strengthened, that healthcare systems are broken, that an epidemic is looming.

Contrasting the epistemological certainty of statistics against the parlance of management immediately exposes diabetes's capriciousness. If you google the phrase, "things you should never say to a person with diabetes," for example, multiple lists appear detailing the daily annoyances confronted by those who live with the disease. "You'll grow out of it," relays one person of the condition, noting the confusion stemming from the phrase "juvenile" diabetes. Another contributor laments the refrain, "you must have the bad kind," a mysterious colloquialism considering no form of diabetes is without complications. Even seemingly absurd quips make appearances on these lists: "I know all about diabetes. My cat has it!" Feline diabetes, while no walk in the park for the cat, is far less complex than that of its human counterparts. Among the most recurring nuisances reported by those composing the lists were messages that confuse type 1 with type 2: "You just need to eat better and get more exercise," reports one participant. "But you're not fat," writes another. "If you lose ten pounds, you could go off insulin," a blogger remembers with disbelief. Individuals posting the lists acknowledge that most interlocutors are well intentioned, even if their input creates an atmosphere inhospitable to actual care regimens. And while many of the lists do not do a remarkable job of dispelling the shame that tends to accompany comparisons between type 1 and type 2, they do underscore how little many people actually know about diabetes, despite its ubiquity.

When Treichler penned *How to Have Theory in an Epidemic*, her groundbreaking tome about the early years of the AIDS crisis, she noted that even those renderings of HIV/AIDS that were not scientifically "correct" lent insight into the ways medical phenomena are deciphered. Haitians, for example, were never disproportionate carriers of HIV, despite being one of the original "four H" risk groups.[15] But their inclusion in that classification revealed much about how the United States conceived the relationship among race (and by extension racism), nationalism, and disease. AIDS was not, we can assume, a punishment from above, but suggesting that a deity was disciplining gay people influenced the response to HIV for decades in places of worship that extended from the Vatican to churches in the American South. Put simply, there is no separating medical epistemologies from their cultural domains. Before moving on to the vast forms diabetes management adopts, which can be as fanciful and bizarre as Treichler's list for AIDS, I briefly outline the types of diabetes that are predominant in the medical sphere, even if such designations are not themselves always semiotically stable.

Typologies of Diabetes

Diabetes tends to be distinguished in three ways: type 1, type 2, and gestational. Type 1, previously referred to as "juvenile" diabetes, is an autoimmune disease that strikes suddenly and develops rapidly. Once associated with youth, type 1 is now signified without the prefix of "juvenile" because it can manifest at any time during the life span and most people who have it are not children.[16] Although the precise cause of type 1 diabetes is a mystery, it is ordinarily accepted that the immune system mistakenly attacks and destroys the insulin-producing beta cells of the pancreas. It is not fully understood why the body misrecognizes itself, though scientists have speculated everything from a viral intruder to genetic predispositions, to some combination thereof.[17] As a result, the pancreas is unable to regulate glucose levels, neither producing insulin nor recognizing when trace amounts of sugar are needed to keep a body in motion. Without insulin, the endocrine system is unable to transform sugar into glucose, which cells depend on for energy. As such, insulin must be injected into the skin by a mechanical pump or a needle. Insulin is not without its annoyances. Take too much and blood sugar will drop dramatically, producing a condition called hypoglycemia that can cause fainting, unconsciousness, or rarely, a diabetic coma. Conversely, too little insulin spurs hyperglycemia and the accompanying effects of ketoacidosis. There is no cure for type 1 diabetes, so insulin injections are indispensable to survival. This is the more unstable and hence fantastic form of diabetes seen in films such as *The Panic Room* and *Steel Magnolias*.[18] The fact that type 1 is largely invisible—both interpersonally and in the public sphere—likely contributes to the idea that it can be casually managed.

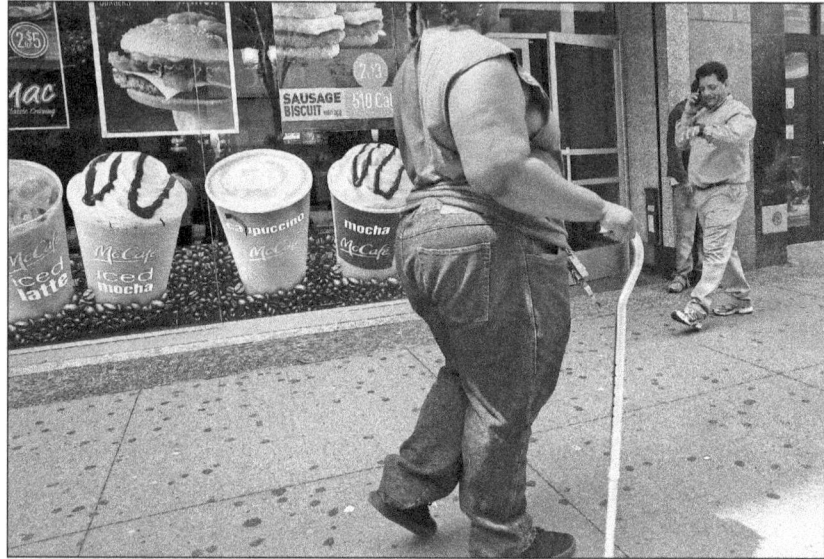

Figure 1.1. Image featured in *The Independent* article, "Diabetes Could 'Bankrupt the NHS' After 60% Rise in Number of Diabetes Cases, Charity Warns," August 16, 2015. Spencer Platt/Getty Images News/Getty Images.

Type 2 diabetes, on the other hand, is often diagnosed in people who are older and sometimes overweight. Whereas type 1 is characterized by a lack of insulin, people with type 2 either do not produce enough insulin or their cells lose sensitivity to insulin and ignore it.[19] This form of diabetes is typically controlled through oral medication, although type 2 can also necessitate insulin if the pancreas disengages fully from its normal functions. Type 2 diabetes constitutes about 90 percent of all cases and is most lethal because it can remain undetected for years. Once associated with wealth and whiteness, type 2 diabetes has evolved in disparaging fashion to be affiliated with minority and low-income communities. A metonymic correlation is frequently crafted in media outlets among race, consumption, and the moral failings of not rigorously maintaining the body. A widely circulated photo of an African American woman whose head is cropped out of the frame and who is utilizing a cane as she walks past a McDonald's points to the problematic representations that are imparted about type 2 diabetes. The line of sugary drinks and high-calorie meals metaphorically dissolves into the woman's body, drawing a straight line between consumption, responsibility, and disability. And while the products are on full display, the woman herself is dehumanized: She literally has no head. As such, all that audiences can presume to know about her identity is made in association with the visual referents around her. When coupled with the headline, "Diabetes Could 'Bankrupt the NHS' After 60% Rise in Number of Diabetes Cases, Charity Warns," this woman's control is imagined to be out of bounds, affecting not simply her, but the body politic as a whole.

Culturally then, these two forms of diabetes are distinct because of the blame assigned to people with type 2.[20] As noted earlier, narratives commonly adopt an accusatory tone, contending that if a person simply would have eaten less, managed their diet, or exercised more, they would not be struggling physically and emotionally. Whereas people with type 1 diabetes have an onset period of several weeks, signaling the decreased capacity of the pancreas, type 2 develops at a glacial pace, leaving most cases undetected for years. As a result, in the cultural schema of diabetes, people with type 1 are widely cast as victims, while those with type 2 are positioned as deserving of this outcome because of their overconsumption. Although people with type 2 sometimes have more control over their body, it is an oversimplification to assert that there is a single causal agent of diabetes or that it can be easily remedied. It is also a mistake to assert that all people who are classified as overweight will develop diabetes, as the vast majority of people, including those labeled obese, never will.[21] Chapter 2 deals explicitly with this stratification system, examining the ways shame shapes surveillance and limits productive intervention strategies for addressing diabetes rates.

Diabetes's denominations are not wholly structured around the stark binary between types 1 and 2. As scientific understandings of the endocrine system have evolved, so too has the volatile and fluid role of glucose in the body. Many people, for example, live with latent autoimmune diabetes in adults (LADA), which is sometimes referred to as type 1.5 diabetes. In LADA, the presence of antibodies negatively engaging the body exists, as it does with type 1, but the onset period is slower. The pancreas is still producing some insulin, but injections are customarily needed within six years. Still other people live with forms of monogenic diabetes, also known as mature onset diabetes of the young (MODY). This rendition of diabetes is typically diagnosed in people younger than 25 who experience (often undetectable) hyperglycemia that never progresses toward ketoacidosis. Researchers have also begun studying the connection between Alzheimer's disease and insulin resistance, sometimes referring to it as "type 3" diabetes. Scientists theorize that insulin deficiency to the brain causes neurodegeneration that catalyzes Alzheimer's. The relationship between Alzheimer's and diabetes has been circulating in medical circles for at least a decade and could help to advance knowledge about the biochemical exchanges between diabetes and various parts of the body. From a cultural perspective, it is imperative that we monitor the rhetorical development of "type 3" diabetes and its potential affinities with type 2. It is entirely possible that blame might be foisted on to people with Alzheimer's for their diagnosis, as it has for other variants of diabetes. For better or for worse, new forms of knowledge are always articulated to previous epistemological tendencies that rest outside the confines of medical taxonomies.

Finally, although gestational diabetes receives the least amount of attention in this text, it certainly deserves mention. The disciplining that occurs during pregnancy, especially for women with any trace of sugar irregularity, promulgates significant parallels with rhetorics of excess, shame, and projections of the productive body. The American Diabetes Association reports that doctors do not know why some women develop gestational diabetes and others do not. Scientists hypothesize that hormones produced by the placenta spark insulin resistance, initiating hyperglycemia in expectant mothers. The condition tends to be temporary and does not stay with women after they give birth. Gestational diabetes can create problems for the fetus (including a higher risk for type 2 diabetes later in life) but is ordinarily treatable. Nonetheless, meaningful intersections can be found between diabetes and pregnancy: Pregnancy is perennially couched in terms related to personal responsibility and the role of the mother as a "protector" above all other things. Likewise, women's bodies are monitored during pregnancy and they are judged when they eat the "wrong" foods, drink any trace of alcohol, or consume caffeine. The body is rigorously surveyed, not necessarily by the mother herself, but by loved ones, acquaintances, and even strangers. Moralizers regularly police the bodies of pregnant women and people with diabetes, and combining them produces an ominous form of public supervision.

The disciplinary tendencies that accompany diabetes highlight the degree to which management has been couched in and grounded by neoliberal conceptions of agentic subjects and their relationship to biopolitical performances of governmentality. That is, undergirding the logic of diabetes care regimens, there is an assumption of a person who has the ability to make particular, if undefined, choices in order to achieve an abstract goal of control. These impressions of diabetes have been given much attention in studies that focus on the clinic, a site that not only has generated an impressive amount of medical data, but one that has nurtured diabetes's public character and the lexicon we tend to adopt when discussing it. Iterations of management as a public disease do not rest apart from those that are situated in the microcosm of the clinic. Rather, they are mutually informative, offering insights into the development of public narratives about diabetes and its disparate forms.

Management: A Paradigm of Personal Agency

In the early twentieth century, chronic medical conditions killed approximately one-fifth of the US population.[22] People were more likely to die from pneumonia, tuberculosis, or diarrhea than they were from diseases such as diabetes. Thanks to advances in science and medicine, many of the environmental and infectious agents that once plagued us have been eradicated, helping to extend the human life span by nearly three decades. As a result, chronic conditions now claim the lives of nearly 80 percent of the population.[23] This dramatic transformation in public heath necessitated a vocabulary for contending with the everyday consequences of chronic diseases, and there is no paradigm more ubiquitous than that of "management." Turn on the television and you're bound to see commercials for COPD medications that spotlight management as a central concern.[24] Anti-obesity campaigns continually stress exercise regimens and dietary management to maintain wellness.[25] Management is invoked in public rhetorics dealing with depression, diabetes, epilepsy, asthma, fibromyalgia, coronary artery disease, hemophilia, chronic fatigue syndrome, and erectile dysfunction.[26] Even diseases that were once classified as exclusively infectious, such as HIV, are now regarded as chronic and manageable.[27]

The amalgamation of conditions outlined above illustrates the fungible nature of management and its plasticity in public rhetorics about health and medicine. In each instance, the framework of management endows patients as recipients of technological knowledge and medical aptitude. Medical epistemologies of the past envisioned the body as a machine in need of repair and bestowed the locus of expertise to physicians who could rehabilitate it. Today's conceptions of management, conversely, assign direct agency to people living with disease.[28] Such regimens permit those who know their bodies best to steer quotidian treatments and enhance their quality of life, as long as they have access to lifesaving resources to stay well. Zoltan Majdik and Carrie Ann Platt argue that management fosters "a perspective that connects potential loci of action and choice to domains lay audiences feel comfortable with and competent in."[29] The expertise imparted to individuals, however, can create equally daunting problems. Many scholars have warned that management incites an obligation to conform to the imperatives of public health mandates and those who craft them.[30] Patients are increasingly responsible for adopting the knowledge furnished by medical and state authorities, performatively rehearsing scripts that appear self-evident in their execution and effect.

Blurring the boundaries of medical aptitude between patient and physician suggests management is not easily studied using only biopolitical theories of governmentality or neoliberal projections of personal agency, even though many works engage one or both of these to investigate management's conceptual scope. Michel Foucault's works on discipline and surveillance are certainly useful for contemplating the reach of medical norms, but so too are his notions of resistance, technologies of the self, and the development of moral personhood. Attempting to determine where the clinic door ends and the currents of everyday life begin is a knot that is not easily untangled. William Donnelly's call for "clinical arts" and Arthur Kleinman's push for "meaning-centered" notions of care both reflect the ongoing conceptual messiness of communicating about illness by acknowledging the reach of medicine into quotidian practices without relinquishing the ways people appropriate, articulate, nuance, and omit medical directives from daily routines.[31] In a similar vein, Peter Conrad has famously noted the ascendance of medicalization, a process that seeks to impart increased individual control over disparate conditions through technological and pharmaceutical intervention.[32] Even as diabetes is assuredly a medical reality, management has followed the path of medicalization, becoming a catchall for diffuse bodily treatments and maintenance. Navigating the fictive extremes of structurally determined public health mandates on the one hand, and patients with unfettered agency to make "the correct" choices on the other, requires a focus on the meaning-making practices of people with diabetes and the unexpected, sometimes convoluted, ways they process ideas associated with management. Numerous scholars have attempted to gauge these formations by probing one particularly rich site: the clinic.

Guided by questions of structure and agency, researchers have focused on the scene of the clinic and the interactivity between clinicians and patients to ascertain management's benefits and deficiencies. These literatures, which draw provocative conclusions, tend to emphasize the operative force of the clinic in the lives of people with diabetes. Mary Specker Stone, for instance, scrutinized patient empowerment strategies by ruminating on the ways the body of a person with diabetes shifts from an active agent to a passive part of the medical scene, in the process actualizing directives that undermine patient agency.[33] Echoing Foucault, she finds that those with diabetes "carry a bit of the clinic" wherever they go.[34] Anthropologist Steve Ferzacca found that both physicians and patients embrace mutual commitments to abstract ideals such as discipline and health, but observed that patients articulated these shared notions to unconventional and idiosyncratic regimens that were rarely effective.[35] Mol notes the contradictions that stem from clinical encounters, arguing that physicians must balance a delicate situation, providing spaces for sadness and reflection, but also encouraging patients by emphasizing the power of modern treatments to foster a healthy life.[36] Still other scholars have found that ethnic differences have the effect of fortifying dominant medical models by isolating anything not intelligible to doctors as a matter of cultural, and not institutional, shortcomings.[37] The focus on the clinic has produced much needed research, but it comes at the risk of cementing conceptions of health and well-being in institutional locations at the expense of enclaves where knowledge is produced and circulated in equal measure.[38] Of course, there is good reason for this. The clinic provides a judicious and workable realm of study, where conclusions can be drawn with some degree of verifiable evidence and data that can be replicated.

Although medical advancements have enabled patients to assert more control over their conditions, providing them with strategies for maintaining wellness, the ways patient agency has been popularly imagined evokes its own anomalies. Lora Arduser has detailed the necessity to disarticulate patient agency from problematic frames such as "compliance" and move toward relationships that speak to the nuances of self-care.[39] Patients can be enabled by agentic practices, but such strategies can produce as many limitations as they do possibilities for being healthy. For instance, the moving target of perfect control for people with diabetes, represented by the idealized glucose reading of 90, illustrates the recalcitrance of focusing exclusively on a narrowed goal for success. The injection of insulin is necessary for the stabilization of blood sugar levels. But, the substance also triggers experiences that are regarded as unmanageable. In their study of the semiotics of the term hypoglycemia, Mol and John Law captured the tensions that exist between methods of control with insulin and the ways people make sense of diabetes. Paradoxically, hypoglycemia is something that transpires *because of control*, not in spite of it.[40] Rigorous regulation offers the prospects of longevity, but it comes at the cost of feeling ceaselessly out of sorts if hypoglycemia persists. It can also instigate neurological problems if sugar is regularly denied to the brain. Hypoglycemia incites harm, even as taking insulin is customarily regarded as promoting *stability* in blood sugar. Many insulin-dependent people can recall instances when they underdosed for the sake of not initiating hypoglycemia in a public setting, perhaps when giving a presentation or driving long distances on the highway. The contingent character of disease necessarily means that compromising and sometimes counterintuitive decisions need to be made. As David Morris reflects, disease and illness "always contain deeply practical imperatives: Something must be *done*, often quickly and with imperfect knowledge."[41] Translating medical ideals into lived praxis is not easily accomplished, and failures tend to be attributed to individuals and not the internal contradictions of management.

The moral imperative to conform to health strategies and remain robust is usually strong among those managing chronic conditions, even when life's entanglements are unrecognized by people making judgments about such efforts. As a nurse practitioner who specializes in diabetes once told me, the hardest part of her job was convincing patients that having atypical blood sugars did not make them bad people. Management's individuation can generate feelings of isolation and helplessness just as much as empowerment and control.[42] When people with diabetes do not conform to numerical averages and social models of productivity, they are frequently left devastated by the results, particularly if blood sugar averages are persistently erratic. Control becomes closely aligned with positive values, "described as a marker of virtue, will, maturity, and autonomy; declining to control it indicated laziness, gluttony, or, simply, ignorance."[43] This resonates with the observations of disability scholars who find that any digression from the exalted norms of bodily productivity in a postindustrial society will lead to charges of dysfunction.[44] The National Institute of Mental Health (NIMH) reports that people with diabetes are twice as likely to experience depression because of management fatigue and feelings of worthlessness.[45] The NIMH conveys that stigma is strong for those who are perceived by themselves and others as not managing the body properly, evoking both physical and emotional turmoil. How individuals *should* care for themselves is well known among people with diabetes, but achieving health ideals can be more daunting than is sometimes imagined. Mol reminds us that what constitutes "improvement" in diabetes care is not always transparent. "Traditionally," she argues, "health was the ultimate goal of health care. These days it rarely is. In chronic diseases health is beyond reach, and it has been replaced by the ideal of a 'good life.' But what counts as a 'good life' is neither clear nor fixed."[46] The individuation of disease and the moral implications engendered by management continually, if inadvertently, vacate the adverse aspects of disease in idiosyncratic instances.

Scrutinizing management heralds its own internal tension: We cannot confidently assert that management rhetorics deterministically structure life for people with diabetes, but neither can we assume that people with diabetes have complete agency over their disease at all times. On the one hand, those extolling the virtues of management habitually, if unintentionally, contend that people are granted "equal status as citizens," overlooking structural disparities lurking in the laudable goals of healthy living.[47] On the other hand, institutional directives do not perform a necessitarianism that guides every action of the patient. Despite stigma, shame, and the debilitating aspects of management, people find ways to make do and—consciously or not—evade overly prescriptive demands. This negotiation presents an important balance, especially when some studies have found that over-managing diabetes can be harmful. Diabetes requires a strong sense of prudence. It demands people to decipher the contours of disease by applying broad principles to specific situations. Such common sense is not easily developed and often requires years of arbitration between medical necessity and lived reality. As another health educator imparted to me when I was first diagnosed, people with diabetes must be cautious about the advice given by others—everyone thinks they know how to manage diabetes. A strong sense of what works for your body, and what does not, becomes imperative for survival. A prudential approach to care avoids generalizations that celebrate a machinist body or that reflect the worst impulses of the scientific method.

This attention to judgment, which demands that patients refine fundamental principles for situated action, is also instructive in that it suggests the varied nature of diabetes and allows us to resist easy conclusions about both etiology and management regimens. People with diabetes have discrepant experiences with the condition, and those lived realities foreground multiplicitous aspects of disease. Management always has the potential to slide into conceptual singularity. But a narrowed and ill-conceived conception of management, often adopted by people not in the medical sphere, can be deleterious when it is unreflectively applied across bodies and situations. Take something as simple as the stark classification system between types 1 and 2 diabetes. Commonsense renderings of the disease might tell us that people with type 1 developed the condition as children and type 2 later in life. And sometimes this is the case. Yet this assumption can be equally problematic. On at least one occasion I have had to convince a physician that I did not live with type 2 diabetes. The fact that I was diagnosed later in life led him to conclude that I had type 2 and that I might not need insulin. Age became a reductive marker for my disease, rather than the mysterious catalyst that actually triggered its onset. The meaning-making process underwriting management sometimes requires patients to revisit and rehearse the most basic aspects of living with a chronic disease. Those with diabetes must possess a surprising degree of social sagacity in order to stay well. Presumed understandings of diabetes can produce as many obstacles to care as they do opportunities for identification and, in the process, exacerbate the schism between public interpretations of management and the prudent skills honed by people with the condition.

Before continuing, it should be noted that the focus on the clinic also suggests, and recurrently obscures, the economic imperatives that accompany diabetes. Just as breast cancer screenings sought to save multinational corporations millions, so too have patient-educational endeavors that deal explicitly with diabetes.[48] Writing in the late 1990s, Stone observed that many HMOs and PPOs incentivized patient "empowerment" because prevention was a cost saver. Like breast cancer programs, empowerment campaigns rarely address the root causes of diabetes, be it systemic poverty, environmental hazards, or a lack of food choices. Not surprisingly, these corporate strategies have rarely translated into economic advantages for people with diabetes. Peter Conrad and Rochelle Kern rightfully observe that "very few of our resources are invested in 'health care'—that is, in *prevention* of disease and illness. Yet, with the decrease in infectious disease and the subsequent increase in chronic disease, prevention is becoming ever more important to our nation's overall health and would probably prove more cost effective- than [reactionary] 'medical care.'"[49] Management here is conceptually offensive and defensive, acting as a driving force for national budgets and personal health, respectively. Although the ACA has given more US citizens access to health care than ever before, it still falls short of universal coverage that would benefit all people with chronic conditions. As of this writing, there is no guarantee that the law will be left intact at all.

Economic considerations present yet another way diabetes might be made intelligible by emphasizing the high cost of being ill and the systemic disadvantages it perpetuates, but seldom do these themes find a home in public culture. People with type 1 diabetes face more economic hardship than those without because of the lifelong consequences of a condition that often begins in childhood. Monthly costs vary depending on the kind of diabetes one has and its severity, but some estimates put expenses at up to $1,000 a month.[50] Along with the burden of medical costs, those with the disease have lower lifetime earnings and fewer job prospects than those without it. People with type 1 earn approximately $160,000 less in their lifetimes than those without the disease because they are less likely to finish high school, attend college, or land a good job. Of course, college might not be possible because of financial difficulty from having a chronic condition in a country that lacks an adequate single-payer system. The *New York Times* reports, "One driving force . . . may be the difficulty in balancing school or job demands with the management of a chronic disease. Employers may also be less likely to hire someone with diabetes because they fear they will take more sick days or be less productive or more of an insurance burden than other workers."[51] These structural concerns do not indicate all is lost, but they do imply that much work remains to ensure that people are financially, legally, and medically protected from such harms.

The remainder of this chapter looks beyond the clinic, to cultural mediations of diabetes management. In some ways, I have been operating outside the walls of the clinic for much of this chapter, pointing to interpersonal interactions, economic longevity, and prudent approaches to care. Even a familiar word like "diabetic" hints at the sociality of disease, literally joining personhood and illness in its utterance. The increasingly common "people with diabetes," conversely, gives presence to the human element of disease, subtly resituating notions of power, subjectivity, and agency. Even in this more progressive representation of disease, it is important to remember that illnesses are not uniform across bodies, and, as queer scholarship reminds us, normativities are not always based on actually normative practices.[52] Just as monogamy is the normative ideal and not always the norm, decrees about how diabetes should be managed might stand in contradistinction to the lived realities of people with diabetes. Anselm Strauss has observed that an abundance of information "generally ignores a basic aspect of chronic illness—how to deal with such ailments in terms that are *social*—not simply medical."[53] Conrad echoes these sentiments when he argues, "it has long been observed that the clinical gaze or the clinical medical model focuses on the individual rather than the social context."[54] Considerations of locality, tradition, and configurations of management can revise suppositions about patient compliance—a loaded phrase if ever there was one—and bestow focus on power structures, norms, and the resources available to make informed decisions. Diabetes is located in a "complex field of power" and its materialization in specific contexts affects how it is recognized among publics.[55] The ways diabetes is made intelligible—as epidemic, as fatal, as the new technological frontier—divulges attitudes about everything from personal directives to institutional interventions that execute disease management.

I want to reiterate that I am not arguing against the medical management of diabetes. Rather, I want management to be engaged as a dense and politically fraught concept that is not only clinical, but cultural. Not simply individual, but social. Not a singular expression, but a series of diverse conventions. If it is true, as thinkers such as Emily Martin attest, that culture and medicine are always already intertwined, then it would prove expedient to expand our purview of management's materializations.[56] I do so in what follows by emphasizing various instantiations of diabetes in the public sphere, glancing at sites where meaning-making happens outside of a medical context, even if that apparatus is always informing the constitution of disease. In the tradition of cultural studies, management is imagined here as a key word that enlivens and makes present one element of Raymond Williams's ephemeral "structure of feeling" for people living with diabetes.[57] I survey an array of artifacts to ascertain management's complex cultural character and offer texture to staid medical renderings of diabetes.

Medical Humanities and the Art of Management

The epigraphs to this chapter share a number of commonalities that speak to the embodied nature of knowledge production and the performative repertoires that transform abstractions into lived practices. Each of them depicts a peripatetic actor, one who walks to make the strange familiar. *Phaedrus* is one of the few dialogues in Plato's canon where his heroine leaves the walls of Athens, signaling the unusual nature of the text and metaphorically encapsulating the dangers of rhetoric's promiscuous circulation outside the bounds of discreet contexts. Anzaldúa is likewise on an excursion, consumed by the beauty and stench of nature, hoping her stroll will draw inspiration for the very exercise Plato suspiciously castigates. Socrates scans the plane trees for cicadas; Anzaldúa the cypress trees that exist harmoniously with the pelicans. They are both preoccupied with invention and spiritual creativity, a yearning for revelations that spring from engagements with the environment, an interlocutor, and oneself. They achieve philosophical clarity through methodological messiness. Plato seeks to rethink the postulates of rhetoric and love; Anzaldúa narrates a morning in her life to craft a poetics of illness in all its inglorious forms.

Plato and Anzaldúa offer alternative paths for contemplating the process of knowledge creation, be it about disease or philosophy or love, and the fruitful rewards of digressing from socially sanctified practices. Their musings invite us to deliberate anew about how diabetes's public persona might be actualized in ways not often attended to in public culture. This section aspires to perform such labor by joining in the chorus of works that investigate, queer, and complicate traditional maps of health and medicine. Once left to the auspices of the social sciences, studies of health and medicine have vaulted into the center of humanistic research. As Anzaldúa's quote conveys, humanists are not new to such endeavors and have long been captivated by the bewildering nature of the body. Luminaries such as Virginia Woolf, Susan Sontag, Audre Lorde, and Eve Kosofsky Sedgwick are among the many thinkers who have sought to trace the amorphous silhouettes of disease. Today these works are taught globally to students in courses focused on health and medicine, especially in the United States, where medical humanities programs have exploded. The number of health humanities programs for undergraduates has quadrupled since 2000, providing opportunities to study the scope and influence of medicine in disparate realms of life.[58] This popularity stems in part from the enhanced focus on interdisciplinarity in higher education. So-called cluster hires, for example, have been implemented by administrators to focus research programs and brand their institutions with specializations that deliver grant money. These clusters often incorporate faculty from medical schools and encourage topics that revolve around health and wellness. When I was in residence at the University of Iowa, for example, a cluster hire was approved by the provost to explore the subject of obesity, and diabetes research was a key element of that work. These programs point to the economic imperatives of the modern university, which were crystallized during the financial crisis of the late aughts. As Belinda Jack has succinctly argued, "There's money in medicine and not so much in the humanities."[59] On a more optimistic note, there is also no denying that there has long existed a dynamic relationship among pedagogy, scholarship, and advocacy in the humanistic investigation of health and medicine. After all, what would AIDS look like without activism? Indeed, what would queer theory look like without studies of HIV/AIDS? What would reproductive rights be without feminist critiques of science? How remiss would the designation of "mental health" be if reduced to definitions outlined by the *Diagnostic and Statistical Manual of Mental Disorders* (DSM) and without the correctives found in art, music, and literature? The humanities elucidate the fixations and deficiencies of clinical perspectives and highlight the generative possibilities of worldmaking among those living with diabetes. The objects of study and methodologies pertinent to the humanities permit a robust examination of the political climates in which knowledge is conceived.[60] The power relations that privilege some bodies over others might give prominence to questions of disability, race, gender, and sexuality that are occasionally lost in objective renditions of science, even as they are fundamental to the inquiries being performed.

Management, then, is not best engaged as a purely medical heuristic. Rather, we might treat management as an intrinsically rhetorical construct that is best studied by spotlighting ecologies of context, the negotiation of meaning-making across publics, and the mystifying complications that escort the circulation and reception of ideas about its functions. There is no shortage of scholarship, from the sciences to the humanities, illustrating that knowledge production is not an inherently impartial process but one underwritten by the realm of human affairs.[61] Skeptics of scientific objectivity who are suspicious of nominal claims to neutrality have repeatedly dissected normative medical assumptions to discern how culture both enables and restricts interpretive schemas for assessing health expectations.[62] The words used to describe "natural" phenomena matter. The contexts in which those words are used matter. The bodies putting those words into discourse matter. Critical heuristics that focus on the intricacies of meaning-making processes can yield valuable insights about health, identity, and power.

As a scholar who is indebted to the fields of cultural studies, feminism, and queer theory, I accord much consideration to the norms that guide the intelligibility of bodies, the stigma that marks people with disease as polluted or impure, and the symbolic possibilities for public activism. The inclination toward social change strikes me as particularly relevant to this project because diabetes is so rarely treated as an object or effect of political power structures. Privileging the voices and experiences of those who live with diabetes can offer matchless rejoinders to public scripts that overlook diabetes's more unconventional, though no less critical, forms. For example, a posting on the widely utilized tudiabetes.com by a blogger who uses the alias "queer diabetic for universal healthcare" illustrates how meanings not typically foregrounded in the public sphere can subtly shift attitudes in productive fashion. Centralizing an intersection that I have not often come across, she asks: "how exactly are queerness and diabetes connected for you?" Her points are worth relaying in full, reproduced here as they are in the forum. She reports:

-im queer and diabetic. they both exist in me and make me who i am. the simple presence of queer diabetics makes them related.
-i have felt shame and pride at different times about being both queer and diabetic.
-i constantly have to come out as queer and diabetic. the process of coming out always reminds me of my otherness, my deviation from normal, which reminds me of unearned privilege (mine and others) and the subsequent inherent discrimination and oppression created in society. the need to come out also reminds me that (good) health and (hetero)sexuality are constantly presumed. and that is inherently homophobic, diabetaphobic, and ableist.
-im queer and i fight for queer liberation in the streets. but im afraid to get arrested and detained without sugar, insulin, test strips. shouldnt the queer liberation movement be flexible enough to make it safe for me to participate? shouldnt i still be able to be a "hardcore activist" without going into a coma?
-im diabetic and i want a cure, goddammit. would kid-friendly type 1 groups want me to join them in the search and fundraising if they knew about how i have sex? would they be willing to risk their benign-wholesome-white-family/friendly-we-didnt-do-anything-wrong image for my liberation? why not? their fear, my fear must be tied.
-what good is a cure if only rich folks with jobs and health insurance and money can afford it?

-what good is liberation if only some people are allowed to be free?
-what good does it do to "dismantle the police state" if the liberators police and judge our bodies, our medical decisions, our food choices, our worth (based on our ability)?
-i need my meds. i need health insurance. i need love. i need respect & acceptance for my full self.

Management here necessitates health care, medicine, and healthy food choices. But it also demands publics that are sensitive to privilege and marginalization, freedom from fear, mental wellness related to sexual acceptance, and the recognition of one's personhood. The blogger's list posits not simply an arduous subject position, but a queer positionality situated by norms of capitalism, white middle-class respectability politics, and the constant prospects of danger (both internal and external) to her body. Her goal is not simply to tell forumites about diabetes, but to illustrate how we might think about management anew through frames emphasizing activism, queerness, and disability free of social stigma. Such testimonials are vital to expanding the umbrella of management rhetorics and reconfiguring how diabetes might be made knowable.

The incorporation of experience, such as the testimonial above, into studies of health and medicine risks dismissal when litigated through a biomedical model that devalues personal narrative.[63] Certainly, the experiences of one individual will inevitably fail to match wholly with those of others, especially when intersectional considerations of identity and geography are taken into account. Nonetheless, the anecdotal is a reflection of a wider field of discourse that surfaces among a spectrum of possibilities. Foucault was one of the many philosophers of medicine who was "fascinated by the ways experience as well as intellectual inquiry contributed to understanding, the authorization of role, and forms of subjectivity."[64] Giving presence to the lived realities of some bodies over others risks hasty generalizations and reckless universalizing. And, yet, the same can be said for conglomerations of data, abstract theoretical terms, or scientifically essentialized categories. Still, just as Lauren Berlant and Michael Warner explored the power of counter-publics through a now infamous example of erotic vomiting in a Chicago gay bar, so too can a peculiar exemplar or representative anecdote lend insight into the normative forces of culture.[65]

Let's consider the 1989 film *Steel Magnolias*, which probably influenced public perceptions of type 1 diabetes more than any other popular culture artifact in a generation. When I was hospitalized after being diagnosed, a good friend walked into the ICU where I was recovering and declared, with unbridled bravado, "Drink your juice, Shelby!!!" He was referencing a character in the film, played by Julia Roberts, who lives with an especially perilous form of type 1 diabetes. During a pivotal scene in the movie, Shelby experiences a violent bout of hypoglycemia in the salon, Truvy's Beauty Spot, where much of the film takes place. Her mother, played by Sally Field, forces Shelby to drink juice to rectify the medical emergency. Shelby resists the sugary drink and shakes uncontrollably during this portion of the film while her mother infantilizes her in front of the other characters. This intense interaction is perhaps the most iconic scene of the production (the spectacle helped to garner Oscar nominations for both Roberts and Field). Although I take some exception to the exaggerated nature of hypoglycemia as it is depicted in the film, it is likely no accident that one of the most common refrains I encounter, part of the "absent archive" of my everyday life, is people believing that juice is the most effective antidote when my blood sugar is low.[66] As generative as the film has been to the camp lexicon, it problematically depicts diabetes as an explosive condition, one that is both dangerous and, appropriate to the genre, utterly dramatic.[67] As life-threatening as hypoglycemia may be to people with diabetes, these momentary fluctuations are usually simple to amend and they pass quickly.

This widely consumed and circulated scene is perhaps most problematic because it suggests that people with diabetes are unable to gauge the intractableness of their disease. Shelby is lovable, yes, but also represented as being in serious denial about the permeability of her body. She bickers constantly with her mother about having children, a choice her alluded-to doctors warn against. But this is melodrama, so Shelby ultimately pursues pregnancy. This choice, which structures the last third of the film, eventually kills her. Of course, reading *Steel Magnolias* through a clinical lens of management leads to a pretty transparent conclusion: Diabetes killed Shelby. However, if we take a page from the tudiabetes.com blogger above and shift our perspective for assessing the narrative, a queer heuristic for exploring management exposes what is perhaps most unsettling about the film: heterosexuality. Throughout the movie Shelby insists that her body is a productive one, vigorously defending the possibility that her diabetes can be overcome. Shelby's compulsive desire for children seems as essential as her need for insulin. Indeed, in a film that champions the queerness of kinship, Shelby's heterosexuality is every bit as volatile and precarious as her diabetes. It is not simply that diabetes could have been managed, it's that Shelby consciously chose to ignore the constraints of her body and insist that she is "normal." Reproductive heterosexuality appears to have killed Shelby every bit as much as her irregular blood sugar did. Historically queer and disabled characters have met unfortunate, if not punitive, ends in Hollywood cinema, and Shelby's non-normative being, regardless of her girl-next-door persona, conclusively defeated her. Articulating management to notions of heterosexuality, in this particular case, alters how illness might be deciphered.

A production like *Steel Magnolias* highlights one of the many ways people might come to process diabetes—their own or others, rightly or wrongly—outside of proscriptive medical appraisals. People formulate interpretations of disease in assorted ways not reducible to the patient-doctor relationship or clinical data. Diabetes is no exception, with the word "management" itself denoting degrees of flexibility and contingency, if not hazard and risk. As I was writing this book I repeatedly encountered accounts of diabetes that were fascinating, surprising, and disturbing. At least two children died when their parents elected prayer as treatment over medicine. A school district prohibited a boy with diabetes from playing baseball, fearing no adults were qualified to address the hypoglycemia he might experience. They also clearly violated the Americans with Disabilities Act when they refused to hire a nurse to accommodate him. On that note, sometimes diabetes is framed as a disability and sometimes not. Public figures such as Mary Tyler Moore, Jay Cutler, Halle Berry, Sonia Sotomayor, and Bret Michaels spring to mind when thinking about diabetes. Their biographies tend to accentuate discipline, transcendence, and redemption over structural barriers and economic hardship. Many young people know what they do about diabetes because of Nick Jonas, who frequently poses shirtless to show off his muscular physique and visually demonstrate that the siphon is being defeated. Others will immediately think of Wilfred Brimley and his slightly divergent pronunciation of the disease. Controversies, both individual and institutional, abounded during this book's production. Media outlets became fascinated with so-called diabulimics, young women who withhold insulin to lose weight and control their sugars. Their narratives of excessive self-control provided a cautionary tale about restraint, allegorizing the ways management can haunt those it is meant to help most. On the other end of the spectrum, as part of a health campaign the New York City Department of Health and Mental Hygiene (DOHMH) circulated a photoshopped image of an African American man who they erroneously posited had lost a leg to diabetes. The image, scrutinized in chapter 5, called into question the ethics of public health and its incessant desire to reach citizens. New drugs, new insulin pump technologies, and the promise of an artificial pancreas came across my screen consistently as I wrote. None of these anecdotes are meant to evacuate the important medical realities of management, only to say that a variety of affects, logics, and emotions come into play when assessing the vivacious character of diabetes and its management. *Managing Diabetes* focuses on a series of case studies in order to ruminate on the divergent ways management is realized in public culture. In what follows, I submit an extended example to conclude this chapter and exemplify how a move away from a clinical perspective might divine insight into the paradoxes and dislocations of diabetes on a level that is cultural every bit as much as it is medical.

The Art of Care

Jen Jacobs is an artist and schoolteacher in New York City living with type 1 diabetes. In her senior year of college, Jacobs began using art as a medium for dealing with chronic disease in ways that were not reducible to medical parlance. Her paintings take as their object of study varying aspects of diabetes management, ranging from the pseudo-realism of insulin vials to the ephemeral, though deeply alarming, effects of hypoglycemia. Each painting portrays some aspect of daily life for those who are insulin-dependent, concentrating on the temptation of sweets, the intrusive questions asked by acquaintances, and affective bodily responses that lie outside the trappings of language. Taken together, her compositions are collectively generative, pointing to contradictions and incongruities that lurk in the pursuit of personal well-being.

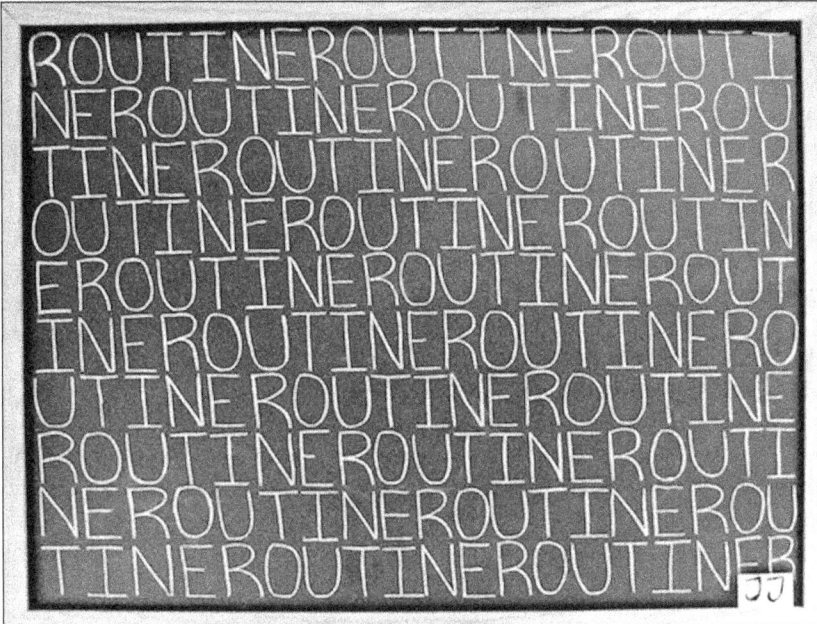

Figure 1.2. Jen Jacobs, "Routine." Used by permission of Jen Jacobs (diabetesart.com).

The contrast between her paintings "Routine" and "Good Morning" challenge the oft-assumed assertions that self-care is transparently plotted. The work depicts a large blackboard (not a surprising choice given Jacobs's occupation) with the word "Routine" written repeatedly over ten lines. The word is recurrently broken up when space runs out at the end of the chalkboard. The reiteration of the word "routine" boldly and appropriately mimics the management regimen it is meant to index. However, due to lack of space on the board, routine is also discrepant in its composition, unsettling the very idea of a direct approach to controlling blood sugar. Despite the lack of coherence suggested in the piece, the entirety of the word "routine" is centered in the middle of the blackboard four lines down. Periodically, it would seem, routine comes together. The creation's purpose appears to convey that to have diabetes is both to perform routine and be caught in its accusational gaze. Management looms large even as one mulls over its simultaneous discontinuities and monotony.

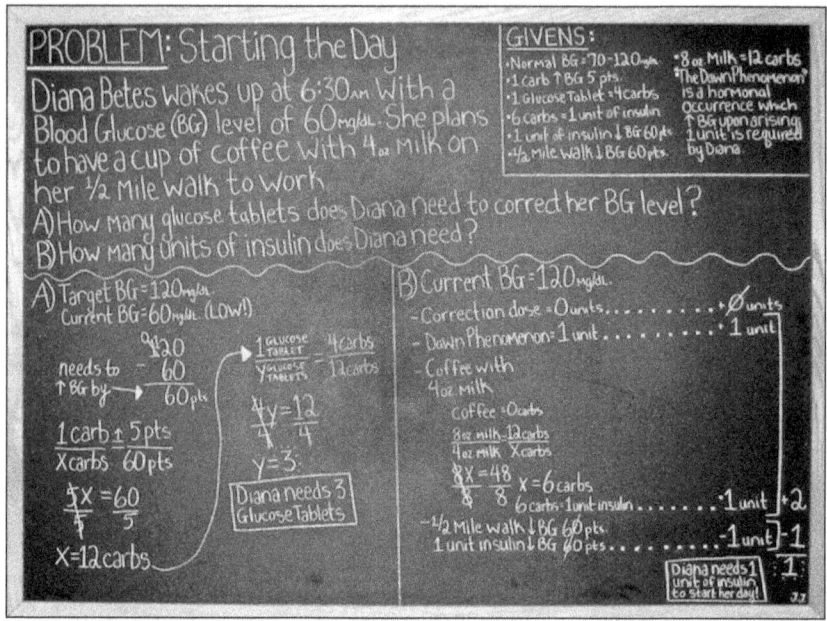

Figure 1.3. Jen Jacobs, "Good Morning." Used by permission of Jen Jacobs (diabetesart.com).

Conversely, her works "Good Morning" and "Every Time I Eat" present the dilemmas of management when the fantasy of habitual technique is disrupted. While "Routine" presents viewers with the idea of persistent, almost dreadful repetition, "Good Morning" probes the intricacies of diabetes management, framing it as a math problem with a preponderance of variables that must be analyzed before eating. Like "Routine," this painting is conceptualized on a chalkboard that insinuates education, critical thinking, and calculation. The problem reads:

> Starting the Day
> Diana Betes wakes up at 6:30 a.m. with a Blood glucose (BG) of 60 ml/dl. She plans to have a cup of coffee with 4 oz. of milk on her ½ mile walk to work.
>
> A) How many glucose tablets does Diana need to correct her BG level?
> B) How many units of insulin does Diana need?

Alongside these words is a segmented table labeled, "Givens," which includes information about her blood sugar targets, the number of carbs in milk and glucose tablets, and the amount of insulin needed to metabolize them. In contrast to "Routine," which is circular despite its periodic breaks, "Good Morning" offers a range of contingencies, some of which will be familiar to observers and others of which may not. The concept of the "Dawn Phenomenon," for example, will likely seem mysterious to many. The dawn effect, as it is also called, is a surge of glucose made naturally by the body in the early morning hours to provide energy for the day ahead. Below the extended math problem are two formulas for calculating how much insulin Diana must administer to herself.

The use of the blackboard in each of these implies a public that is being educated about the tribulations of diabetes. Like many artistic ventures, the work appears to be directed at a universal audience, encouraging patrons to deepen their understandings of the disease, even if it is done through identification with the fictitious Diana Betes and her quandaries. "Good Morning" is not as easily processed as "Routine," as it calls upon viewers to evaluate myriad factors: time, space, consumption,

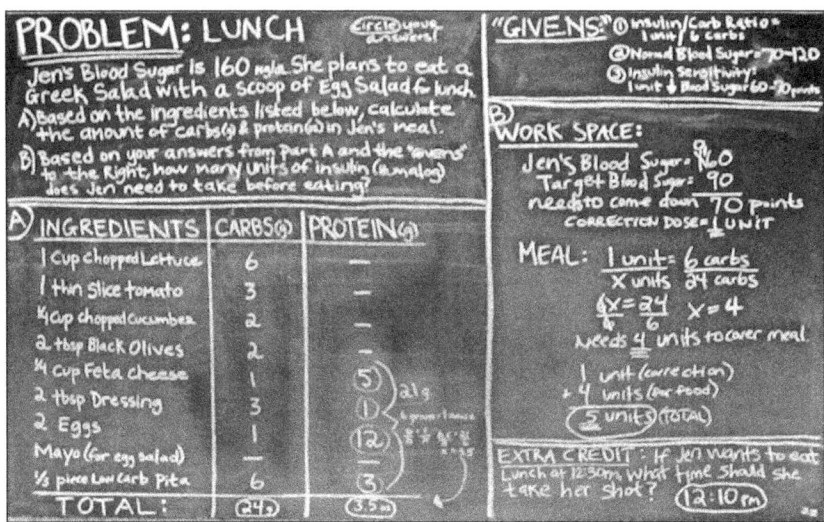

Figure 1.4. Jen Jacobs, "Every Time I Eat." Used by permission of Jen Jacobs (diabetesart.com).

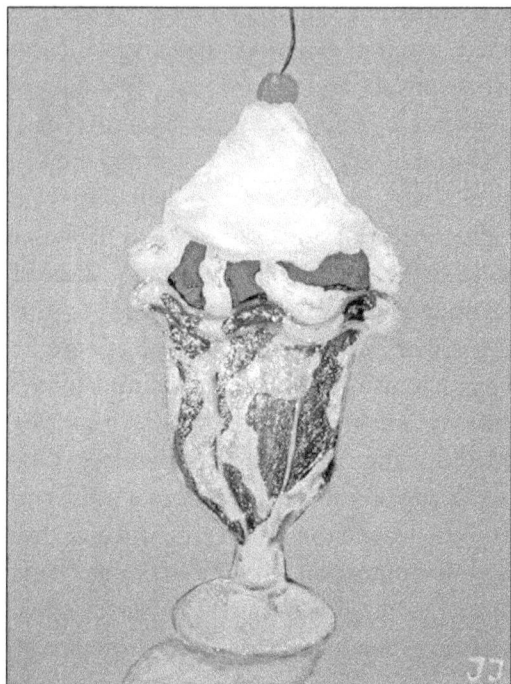

Figure 1.5. Jen Jacobs, "Can You Eat That?" Used by permission of Jen Jacobs (diabetesart.com).

caution, and calculation. Time is a noteworthy theme across Jacobs's work, illustrating repeatedly that people with diabetes are persistently focused on the time of day, the times they need insulin, and the time they have left in this world. Diabetes is, after all, a *chronic* disease, structured around the gradations of the calendar and the gradualism of the clock. In this way, Jacobs's work is astoundingly rhetorical—being concerned with the contingencies of situations as much as they are the universal qualities usually privileged in art.

Being public is a captivating idea in Jacobs's work, giving primacy to the ways diabetes is made relationally intelligible, not simply in the confines of one's home or in the space of the clinic. Both "Can You Eat That?" and "Downtown" highlight the extremes of insulin use, one preoccupying itself with the prospects of hyperglycemia and the other with hypoglycemia. "Can You Eat That?" focuses on a singular object: a large sundae that shimmers on the canvas. Jacobs has noted that her work is sometimes satirical in its impulse. She incorporates humor to deal with the pressures of diabetes, as so many living with the disease do. This painting fits the bill, as any person with diabetes recognizes the absurd exchange this situation immediately invites. The ice cream has multiple layers—hot fudge, caramel, whipped topping, and the proverbial cherry on top. The glass holding the dessert is transparent, but crystalized, representing the very warning that is denoted in the painting's name. The visual material might otherwise be mundane until one realizes that the title is a query directed at a person with diabetes. This is not mere decadence, but also a moment of judgment that is interpretively polysemous. The painting could be depicting an instance of disciplining the diabetic body. It could betoken resistance to other, wiser food choices. It could

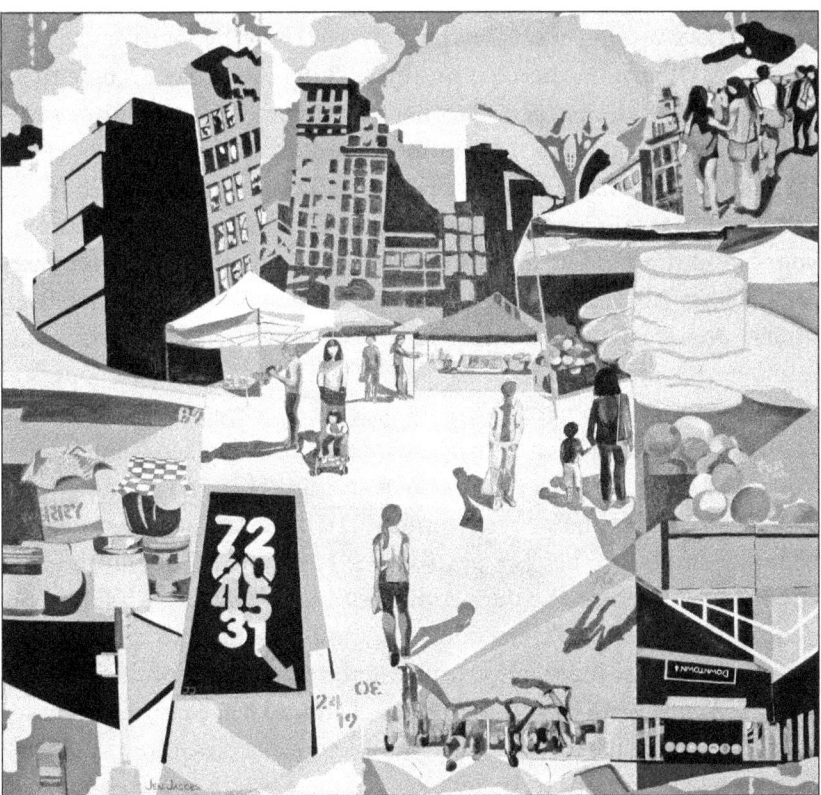

Figure 1.6. Jen Jacobs, "Downtown." Used by permission of Jen Jacobs (diabetesart.com), and the owner, Claude Piche.

reveal anxieties shared among both actors in the interaction—the person posing the question who has no knowledge of what happens next if the person with diabetes elects to eat the ice cream and the burden of being surveyed for the interlocutor with diabetes. The work depicts a moral question as much as it does a medical one, an account that reflects the fleeting but ominous structures that organize the life of someone who is insulin-dependent.

"Downtown" is, to my mind, Jacobs's most compelling painting if only because its abstraction reflects the difficulty of capturing the experience of hypoglycemia. Jacobs's work concocts a memory of her blood sugar descending rapidly at a farmer's market. Like Socrates and Anzaldúa, Jacobs is walking, performing the most ordinary of tasks in an otherwise unremarkable setting, when the hypoglycemia strikes. The feeling of dangerously low blood sugar is experienced differently among people and can have varying effects on the body. For some, hypoglycemia is disorienting. Others may become obstinate. Still others may become tired, weak, giddy, or despondent. Jacobs's painting captures the disorientation created by hypoglycemia, noting the distortions, panic, and anxiety that can materialize if one is in public and others are unaware of the condition. Are you alone? Do you have food or drink that can amplify your blood sugar? How quickly are your levels dropping? The numbers on the board at the bottom left of the painting indicate a quick fall from mild hypoglycemia (the number 72 is low, but still relatively safe) to the number 31, which signifies a dangerous state that can render a person unconscious. The numerals visually slide off of the sign, literally hitting the floor, indicating what is to come if action is not taken immediately. We might expect that Jacobs is one of the figures in the painting (presumably the person next to the numbers) or the entire occurrence might be understood from her perspective. The scene and agent blur into one configuration, where the danger of low blood sugar is both internally and externally present. The shadows on the abstractions stretch in different directions, the buildings are distorted, and the lines discernably not straight. While there is food and drink all around her, confusion persists.

Jacobs's art grants an opportunity to explore diabetes in ways not typically seen in academic literature.[68] Each of these paintings is a snapshot of her life with diabetes that resides outside the realm of the clinic, shining a spotlight on the complications and contradictions of management, the boldness of proclamations about routine, and the nuances that must be addressed to truly apprehend and sympathize with her particular needs and problems. One composition relays the looming desire for sugary food and the self-monitoring it instigates. Another ponders the isolation of disease in the most public of settings. The artist's visual narratives are themselves an important part of life with diabetes for, as Mol tells us, in "the logic of care exchanging stories is a moral activity in and of itself."[69] Jacobs calls attention to balance, temptation, desire, and discipline. The song of the cicadas could be the soundtrack to her gallery.

Chapter Preview

The remainder of this book explores a variety of case studies to provide an overview of diabetes's public personifications. The archive of this volume purposefully works outside strict biomedical renderings of diabetes that limit the scope of how the condition is made intelligible, surveying artifacts as diverse as everyday speech and public health controversies, to ascertain diabetes's amorphous persona. The objects of study in the following chapters are part of a public archive, one composed of media representations, political posturing, and seemingly banal communicative exchanges. The content for each chapter is often mined from news reports but is also composed of congressional testimony, law reviews, and interviews with public health officials. This is not to say that medicine is absent in my archive. Any mention of diabetes carries the rhetorical remainder of that history and I often engage medical reports directly. Following the work of scholars like Berlant, I find that such a prosaic archive exhibits an ordinariness that "requires an intensified critical engagement with what had been undramatically explicit."[70] This archive is itself a form of rhetorical stitching, and I am conscious of the ways my own perspective shapes and narrows management's conceptualization. Like all forms of knowledge creation, my own academic expertise helps to structure the materials being explored here: Two of the chapters are deeply dependent on queer theory and LGBT studies, one on feminist investigations of intersectionality, and all are informed by disability studies in some form.

The chapters are loosely organized around two dialogical pairs that accentuate how diabetes is publicly represented. The first binary situates diabetes as easily managed on the one hand and lethal on the other. The second dyad focuses on the necessity of the individual to overcome the disease, which often stands apart from discourses that call for heightened systemic intervention. These four tropes: effortlessness, fatalism, individual transcendence, and institutional regard, all act as major organizing devices for the next four chapters. I contend in the book's conclusion that these four heuristics blur in discussions of diabetes technologies, elucidating political and cultural obstacles that necessitate contemplation in the decades ahead. As is often the case with academic segmentation, the individual concepts in each chapter bleed into one another as much as they stand apart. The case studies are isolated for the purposes of analytical clarity, aspiring to detail an assortment of themes and figures that constitute diabetes management and the cultural contexts people navigate to make sense of their lives.

As a critic indebted to rhetorical and cultural studies, I have selected the case studies that follow because each elucidates unique qualities about the constitution of diabetes management. Humanities scholars have long utilized particular situations in order to theorize larger cultural trends and social impulses, recognizing that all knowledge creation is inherently contextual and contingent. In this way, the examples that structure each chapter do not strive to make universal claims about the composition of diabetes management. I do not believe diabetes management can be easily reduced to a single theoretical heuristic, even if such ideas sometimes surface in the analysis. Resisting theoretical coherence is not an attempt to delay questions about diabetes management. Rather, it is an attempt to address how diabetes management is constituted in specific instances. The cases studies provide snapshots of how management is regarded in common parlance more than offering totalizing explanations of diabetes's public life. Nonetheless, there is little denying that the dyads selected are ubiquitous in discourses about diabetes. The ideas of ease and fatalism, for example, are widespread in media reports, everyday interpersonal exchanges, and medical monitoring. Indeed, the tension between these two discourses sparked unending consternation when I was first diagnosed. It is not an overstatement to say that this discord provided the initial inspiration for this book.

The next chapter uses as its starting point the controversial analogy "HIV is the new diabetes" to explore how diabetes is cast as an easily managed condition. Medical practitioners who view HIV as a chronic condition have embraced the comparison, but those who cling to the notion that HIV is uncontrollable resist the association. Factions that decry the analogy tend to mischaracterize both diseases by ignoring the commonalities among the conditions and exaggerating the consequences of HIV over those that stem from diabetes. I survey scholarship about HIV's turbulent history to mine the concepts of apocalypse, paranoia, and precarity and scrutinize pockets of resistance to HIV's arrival as a chronic condition. These heuristics detail how HIV has come to be marked as erratic and onerous, while diabetes is situated as a disease readily controlled by pharmaceuticals or personal restraint. Not content with this conclusion, I then invert the pair to appraise how we might reconceptualize our thinking about both conditions, particularly with regard to notions of shame, self-governance, and race.

Chapter 3 looks to the advocacy of the JDRF (formerly the Juvenile Diabetes Research Foundation) and its incessant drive to cure type 1 diabetes. The organization is generally heralded as one of the most successful patient lobby groups in the United States, having raised more than $1 billion for scientific research. The JDRF's most lauded and high-profile event is the Children's Congress, in which dozens of young people with type 1 diabetes descend biennially on Capitol Hill to testify before the US Senate. Unlike chapter 2, which explores the idea that diabetes is easily managed, the JDRF's rhetoric contends that diabetes is deterministically fatal. JDRF youth activists argue that management may prolong life, but no amount of personal care can stave off diabetes's lethal arrival. The somber tone adopted by the advocates creates a melancholic projection of the future, something to which they aspire but may never see. Ultimately, I argue that fatalism has a productive place in management discourse by offering a sense of urgency to the condition to marshal institutional resources. Their pleas also resist notions of self-determination and individual responsibility that tend to characterize uninformed impressions of diabetes.

Supreme Court Justice Sonia Sotomayor and her life with type 1 diabetes are the focus of chapter 4. Sotomayor's confirmation hearings were famously clouded by institutional racism and sexism. She was accused repeatedly of being intemperate, emotional, and illogical in a judicial sphere that prizes circumspection, deliberateness, and collegiality.

Perversely, these prejudices also furnished a backdrop wherein her diabetes could be taken to illustrate her personal restraint. The Obama administration highlighted her lifetime of managing type 1 diabetes as proof of personal control and by extension judicial prudence. This strategic invocation of intersectionality, using a disability to rhetorically "contain" race and gender, was remarkably successful. Press coverage originally posited Sotomayor's diabetes as a reason to withhold confirmation. After the White House released a letter from her doctor affirming that she had "consistent blood sugars better than 98% of diabetics," however, this narrative was reconfigured and her condition was situated as a personal strength that would benefit the nation. Management is figured here as a transcendent mechanism and Sotomayor as a so-called super crip. Diabetes may be omnipresent, but its effects can be superseded so long as the person living with the condition "takes care of themselves." Sotomayor's inspirational story, which took her from a public housing project in the Bronx to the highest court in the land, inadvertently propelled an American Dream narrative that eclipsed structural impediments that complicate diabetes management.

The question of systemic intervention is the focus of chapter 5, which examines institutional efforts to curtail diabetes rates. I look to New York City's controversial diabetes registry program, which requires all labs serving municipality residents to report A1C scores to the Department of Health and Mental Hygiene (DOHMH). The city strove to productively address the crisis facing New Yorkers by providing information and resources to those most in need. However, the government also refused to allow any person to opt out of the program. Privacy advocates argued that the city overreached in its efforts and that diabetes management regimens were best left to individual patients and their physicians. In response, the city situated diabetes as an "epidemic" to justify the program, a contentious move considering that diabetes is not a contagious disease. Despite its limitations, I argue that the "epidemic" frame can act as a catalyst for proffering resources that might aid people living with the disease. I offer a rejoinder to those who assail the registry over privacy concerns, a move that inevitably relegates diabetes to the domestic sphere void of any public character. Not to be overly welcoming of government surveillance, I also weigh the limits of the "epidemic" metaphor by mulling over a controversial DOHMH public service campaign.

That PSA featured an African American actor whose lower leg had been photoshopped out of a picture to imply that uncontrolled blood sugar had made him an amputee and to warn about diabetes's consequences. I find this campaign to be counterproductive to the otherwise laudable goals of government interference because such efforts inspire fear and individual loathing rather than engaging systemic features that give rise to diabetes rates in the first place.

The conclusion of the book, chapter 6, engages the role of the cyborg as an emergent figure for diabetes management. Using Donna Haraway's infamous notion of the cyborg, I focus on the political potential of the concept to move beyond the machinist aspects of cutting-edge diabetes technologies. New innovations such as the artificial pancreas have actualized a rhetoric that foregrounds the "new frontier" of medical advancement, but always with the disclaimer that these breakthroughs do not actually cure diabetes. The incessant focus on the latest technological invention functions to occlude the ways corporations profit from populations made most vulnerable by diabetes. I look to the stalled efforts of developing generic insulins, which have been impeded by a practice known as "evergreening." The development of biosimilars (generic insulins) would drastically reduce the cost of staying well for economically disadvantaged people with diabetes, but this possibility remains evasive more than a century after insulin's discovery. The figure of the cyborg lends an appropriate close to the book, as its ontology accentuates a convergence of frames explored throughout this text: mechanistic ease, encroaching death, worldly transcendence, and institutional might.

2

"HIV Is the New Diabetes"

Analogies of Apathy

"A Day with HIV in America" is a photo campaign designed to combat the stigma of living with HIV as the epidemic marches resolutely through its fourth decade. Sponsored by the nonprofit Test Positive Aware Network (TPAN), the 2011 operation kicked off with a four-minute promotional video featuring an array of advocates of differing races, genders, and ages. One of the spokespeople introduced is a young African American woman who declares that HIV is "the same as having diabetes . . . it's something that you just have to manage." This now common analogy to diabetes did not go unnoticed by the editors at *Queerty*, an online news source for LGBT issues, who singled out the statement and retorted, "But are the speakers in this campaign video correct when they say that HIV is 'the same as having diabetes?' . . . Is HIV really so manageable—or does it come with greater health risks and greater stigmas that should be addressed honestly?"[1] By ending the query with a call for more "honest" deliberation about HIV management, the site indicated to readers that the analogy deserved further scrutiny, if not outright dismissal.

TPAN and *Queerty* are not the first to incite spirited public discussions that engage the role of analogy in the production of medical knowledge. Just as physicians, researchers, and public health officials come to know diseases in comparative fashion, publics generally become acquainted with disease through already sanctioned medical epistemologies. Articulating scientific understandings of disease to accepted cultural frames directs interpretations of communal threats and stimulates possibilities for contemplating treatment and containment. AIDS was famously, if incorrectly, labeled both "gay cancer" and "gay pneumonia." Yellow fever and malaria were frequently studied in tandem because mosquitoes transmit both, even though their causal agents are etiologically distinct. Depending on the literature one reads, fibromyalgia, chronic fatigue syndrome, and depression are variations on a theme or unambiguously dissimilar. More recently, debates rage over analogies likening alcoholism to a disease when it may more accurately correspond to an allergy and be addressed with medication. How we come to know a disease is dependent on a complicated interplay of sociopolitical practices, medical parlance, and the lived proximity of populations to the condition being assessed. Resituating a disease such as HIV from fatal to chronic is accomplished not solely through medicine and technology, then, but by analogically reimagining it alongside conditions that are widely acknowledged as manageable.

The politics of intelligibility underlying comparisons between HIV and diabetes illustrate a conspicuous, though not unprecedented, historical moment for those invested in the shifting logics of conceptualizing chronic conditions. Rhetorically, the analogy works to stabilize the crisis of signification that once marked AIDS, reestablishing life with HIV as habitual rather than volatile. In opposition to the disquieting urgency that once underwrote the incalculability of HIV, the analogy relinquishes the precariousness of AIDS and relocates life with HIV to more secure rhetorical groundings in health and wellness.[2] This movement from a tenuous embodiment to one that renders HIV dormant offers, in the words of Lauren Berlant, a lateral agency that focuses on the maintenance of the body in everyday life.[3] This agency is marked not by the ongoing social trauma that once characterized AIDS narratives, but by a slow and deliberate care of the self. Technological developments for attending to HIV have been as transformative as the virus itself once was, with life expectancy rates for people living with HIV now being roughly equivalent to people who are seronegative. While stigma, depression, and economic disparities remain significant obstacles for many who are living with HIV, advances in medical treatment and prevention have been nothing short of astounding. The comparison to diabetes is not only plausible, but in many cases warranted.

In this chapter I argue that comparisons between HIV and diabetes affect the rhetorical architecture of each disease. The analogy is perhaps most potent because it can be utilized to disrupt the notion that diabetes can be unreflectively managed. Those who believe that HIV emulates features of diabetes tend to focus almost exclusively on the dynamic nature of HIV. Diabetes, conversely, is envisioned as static in the analogy, viewed as treatable with a single pill or with unmindful regimens. A statement such as "HIV is the new diabetes" might be rich with potential but often reduces diabetes to a condition that is effortlessly mastered and in doing so imparts presumptions about the ease of regulating HIV. Not surprisingly, critics sensitive to AIDS's ruinous past assail analogies to diabetes as trivializing the perils of HIV. Those suspicious of the association rehearse familiar scripts about the precarity of HIV even as they cement torpid meanings tied to diabetes, in some cases going as far as to dismiss the reparative promise of actual medical advancements.[4] The alarmist outcry exhibited by platforms such as *Queerty* tell us much about attitudes toward both conditions, accentuating public sentiments about the mutability of HIV and the enigmatic sedimentation of diabetes.

Analogies are complex rhetorical configurations that suggest relations of similitude and difference. The power of analogies lies not in their ability to bestow uncompromising truth claims, but to act as sites of invention for judging something anew. Chaïm Perelman reminds us that etymologically, analogies indicate proportionality, a relation that contributes to the logic (the *logos* implied in the second half of ana*logy*) of argumentative form.[5] The degree to which affinities are accepted depends on a number of factors that are not reducible to discrete variables. As Isaac West has noted, analogies are not best understood as quasi-mathematical formulations; rather, they are dependent on a rich network of contexts, contingencies, and articulations that actualize the potential for knowledge creation in figurative manners apart from encoded meanings.[6] It is the innovative power of analogy that I am most invested in here—looking not to a priori conclusions about one set of experiences at the expense of another, but to the productive possibilities that might be cultivated from the analogy's circulation. In short, if diabetes functions as a stabilizing mechanism for those living with HIV, the latter might also constructively destabilize the sedentary connotations associated with diabetes, reformulating troubling perceptions that glucose irregularities are controlled through sheer force of will. What might the analogy tell us if we asked not how HIV resembles diabetes, but how diabetes—culturally, discursively, and politically—is similar to HIV? I approach this question by scrutinizing the entanglements of the analogy to unsettle the tropes of convenience and placidity that underwrite oversimplified management scripts. In what follows I contemplate how vernacular exchanges about HIV reproduce narrowed understandings of chronic conditions in an era of ongoing endemics. Although the imperative to manage diabetes is at times clarified by the exaggerated nature of HIV, the analogy tends to conceal the former's protean character.

Working from the premise established in the introduction that diabetes is made intelligible in diverse contexts, and that understandings of diabetes are often contradictory, incompatible, and asymmetrical, this chapter looks to the trope of diabetes as a mechanistically governed disease. This figuration stands in sharp contrast to fatalistic rhetorics that personify diabetes as essentially unstable, which is explored in chapter 3. Challenging the credo that diabetes is fundamentally languid, I first examine the ways that HIV has been represented as erratic, immedicable, and destructive. I concoct a rhetorical genealogy of HIV/AIDS from queer theory that imagines HIV's character as cataclysmic, a quality that is captured through the reoccurring figures of apocalypse, paranoia, and precarity. This calamitous narrative delineates shifting interpretations of HIV over time and ultimately provides the grounds for detractors to reject comparisons to diabetes. Next, I turn to the curious case of diabetes being an iterate referent in the emergence of HIV as a manageable condition through the oft-recited refrain that "HIV is the new diabetes." The allusions between HIV and diabetes are increasingly prevalent, shaping the ways each is brought into discourse, even as residual notions of HIV hold tight. I then invert the pair to untidy conventions about signification, stigma, and agency, asking how we might reimagine the ways diabetes is personified. This inversion is not meant to suggest an equivocation of the two diseases or an artificial supplanting of the public health strategies related to one condition onto another. Rather, I contend that the discursive features of HIV/AIDS and its storied history can shape the rhetorical texture of diabetes to complicate the nomenclature of personal sovereignty and medical determinism.

Analogical Parallels? Apocalypse, Paranoia, and Precarity

The evolution of diabetes from a fatal disease to a proxy for surmountable conditions like HIV has been centuries in the making. Diabetes was first observed in ancient times, and situating it as a nominally stable illness is itself a relatively new phenomenon.[7] The "siphoning" of the body suggested in diabetes's etymological root indicates a rapidly deteriorating subject, one who did not have the benefit of time on their side. The mercurial nature of the disease was presumed until the discovery of insulin in the early 1920s, when treatment modalities began to resituate it as a manageable condition. Since that time diabetes, especially type 2, has become associated with passive bodies and states of decay. That typification has had tremendous implications, as it is often falsely assumed that diabetes is easily corralled with medicine and diet changes. Although diabetes has been depicted as both fervently precarious and markedly static, HIV has been couched almost exclusively in the former category. Indeed, HIV's haphazardness has generally prevented its classification as a tractable condition until recently.

Just as diabetes was considered a death sentence for those diagnosed prior to mass-produced insulin, AIDS was generally thought to be fatal before the development of antiretroviral medications. When AIDS surfaced in the early 1980s, it was largely treated as an acute condition whose manifestations overtook the body rapidly. Because AIDS is a syndrome, and not a singular disease, people grappled with varying symptoms that were often strikingly dissimilar. Some people exhibited signs of late-stage HIV infection through Kaposi's sarcoma (a cancer that causes abnormal tissue growth under the skin) and others dealt with rare and aggressive forms of pneumonia, among many other possibilities. Despite this perplexing character, scientists made great headway in addressing AIDS by crafting treatments that stymied the progress of HIV in the body. These breakthroughs were often attributed not only to scientists in the lab, but also to pivotal activist groups such as ACT-UP, who worked tirelessly to raise public awareness, combat government indifference, and demand funding for scientific endeavors. Consequently, as early as 1989 some in the medical community were declaring HIV a chronic condition, even though rates of death from HIV/AIDS climbed steadily through the mid-1990s.[8] These medical interventions were often purposefully obstructed by opportunistic politicians who followed a path of misinformation and homophobia in place of public health strategies that actually saved lives. Efforts toward mainstream treatments were often hamstrung by officials who refused to acknowledge HIV's ravenous effects, media representations that reinforced stereotypes, and deeply entrenched institutional maleficence. Even today, this tumultuous legacy continues to hamper prevention efforts for people of color, transgender people, and those on the lowest rungs of the socioeconomic spectrum.

Medical practitioners, scientists, and public health officials were not the only ones grappling with the dilemmas posed by AIDS. Since the beginning of the crisis, artists, scholars, and journalists had been deciphering the ways AIDS was made intelligible as a cultural referent. Thinkers such as Paula Treichler and Susan Sontag were among the many critics who sought to demystify the ways stigma was reproduced on the bodies of marginalized populations, such as LGBT people, and to chart the analogies that brought AIDS into being.[9] The burgeoning field of queer studies became preoccupied with the role of HIV/AIDS as an ordering force in social movements, in the popular evolution of same-sex marriage, and in domains that ranged from the historical to the theoretical. Although there is little room here to detail the many ways that scholarship on AIDS evolved, the ideas of normativity, abjection, and moral panic came to occupy a significant place in the literature. Importantly, as the years passed, this conceptual reservoir expanded and was eventually employed to scrutinize public discourses about a range of diseases and illnesses not confined to HIV. Eve Kosofsky Sedgwick, for example, taught us much about cancer through queer lenses. Ann Cvetkovich did the same for depression.[10] Entire volumes have been penned about the intersection of disabled bodies and sexuality.[11] Ellis Hanson has noted that queer theory's genealogy with AIDS suggests it was born in disability studies, signaling an activist politics indebted to rhetorical understandings of illness and disease.[12] Likewise, I believe HIV's centrality to queer theory and that canon's focus on normativities, temporalities, subjectivities, and affects can help to illuminate the deep complexity of diabetes's public character. I excavate this queer archive to investigate the resistance to recognizing diabetes as HIV's contemporary medical kin. I look to three paradigms in queer studies that have been used to chart cultural connotations associated with HIV/AIDS—that of apocalyptic rhetoric, the critical exploration of paranoia, and the recent emergence of precarity.

That HIV/AIDS have been imagined as destructive and cumbersome is so well documented that it barely requires mention. The advent of

AIDS catalyzed LGBT counter-publics that variously called for radicalism and institutional reform, systemic transformation, and expanded civil rights. The urgency of AIDS activism was enlivened by slogans such as "Silence = Death" and confrontational art that denounced politicians who sat idle while AIDS buried everyone in its path. The rhetorical dynamism of AIDS exerted a plasticity that supersedes its status as a medical phenomenon. It is not an overstatement to suggest that exchanges about AIDS have been no less complicated to decipher than the syndrome itself. The crisis of meaning that marked AIDS affected everything from judgments about "risky" sexual practices to the consequences of heteronormative national imaginaries. This symbolic volatility, underwritten by institutional failures and the anxieties of futures cut short, gave rise to a rhetoric of insecurity that lives on today. The deaths of thousands of people in the face of government neglect and indifference propelled a sense of despondency and impending doom for those who lived through the epidemic's worst days.

The trope of "apocalypse" is perhaps the longest-standing figure in AIDS's unruly mnemoscape. Apocalypse and its dialogical partner utopia are pervasive in the queer canon, operating as two sides of the same coin to mobilize LGBT publics. The pink triangle and the rainbow flag, for example, are both emblematic of LGBT movements, but it is the more obtrusive and ominous triangle that is ubiquitous in AIDS's legacy.[13] Projections of grief and uncertainty can be found in everything from public art to political manifestos to postmodern theories of identity. Focusing on ACT-UP's imposing visual politics, Thomas Long observed the group's provocative graphics "attempt to assess the tactical and strategic instrumentality of apocalyptic discourse" to arouse rage and action.[14] Peter Dickinson took the relationship between AIDS and apocalypse as a starting point, contending, "the problem with abstract theorizing about AIDS is that it frequently lacks a subject, a body, a corpus, a corpse. This would seem to be even more the case when theorizing AIDS as apocalypse."[15] The AIDS Memorial Quilt, Tony Kushner's polemic *Angels in America*, and Larry Kramer's anthology about the early 1980s titled "Reports from the Holocaust," all point toward apocalyptic impulses that dwelled beneath the socio-production of AIDS.[16]

Despite the dire nature of these predispositions, apocalyptic discourse paradoxically imparts agency to those grappling with crises.

A breakdown in meaning leaves open a void to be filled, an ascription of purpose that allows people to interpret events and act on them accordingly. Scholars note that apocalyptic rhetoric energizes a feeling of control over uncertain conditions, even if this clout is figuratively fashioned in a manner that is not politically practical.[17] Contemporary appropriations of apocalyptic speech rarely follow the formal characteristics born in religious genres. Rather, modern-day "secular" or "civil" forms of apocalypse are derived from historically contingent appropriations of these worldviews for addressing anxieties in the present.[18] A simple phrase like "an impending sense of doom" might capture the spirit of such secular inclinations. The expression lends itself to shifting political needs (such as environmental issues or affective political attachments) more so than it does religious dogmas. Fragmented and formally displaced, tropological appropriations of apocalypse discern the malaise of traditional laws and the breakdown of social orders.[19] As the voices in this chapter decrying the analogy to diabetes exhibit, the apocalyptic highlights a temporal disorientation, where the present both fails to bring the past to "utopic completion" and represents a deterioration of collective goals.[20] Apocalyptic attitudes stress the dissolution of long-standing group practices and the inability to realize communal aspirations. The individuation of privately managing the body solves neither the problems presented by AIDS nor collective neglect, inciting renewed calls for vigilance and care until the epidemic recedes once and for all. As we shall see, these themes surface with regularity in comparisons to diabetes.

Advancements in retroviral therapy and access to life-saving drugs made life with HIV less cumbersome for people in positions of privilege as the millennium passed. The panic and strong motivation to combat AIDS—and with it, homophobia—heralded the feasibility of a prolonged life in what some have hailed as a post-AIDS era. No longer relegated to the margins of the polis or the shadows of scientific neglect, HIV was slowly reconfigured into a chronic condition. To be sure, plenty of barriers continued to disenfranchise those living with HIV. Draconian measures that prohibited those who were HIV-positive from entering the United States remained in place. The criminalization of people with HIV who failed to disclose their status to sex partners was (and to some extent remains) widespread. The economic realities of an incongruent and segregated healthcare system presented institutional obstacles for scores of patients. To this day, fears over HIV contamination continue to prevent men who have sex with men from donating blood.[21] Still, much positive change ensued and queer critics began raising questions about the ways paranoia inflected the tenor of discussions about HIV and, by extension, queer lives.

If apocalypse constitutes one early framework for contemplating the AIDS crisis relevant to the analogy with diabetes, then the tropes of "paranoia" and the "reparative" mark the second. Even as queers had substantive reason to cede some fears about HIV, paranoia continued to unfold with conspiracy theories about genocide, lurid tales of bug chasing and gift giving, and scandalous stories about life on the "down low" in communities of color.[22] In a widely circulated essay, Sedgwick pursued a controversial thesis about a paranoid style that had crept into activist and academic queer work. Using as her starting point the rapid uptake of AIDS conspiracy theories, Sedgwick expressed concern about an intellectual predilection that had lost its critical edge and often reproduced the very structures of oppression that queer scholarship sought to tear down.[23] Sedgwick found that paranoia had come to occupy a daunting presence in queer studies, which sought to expose homophobia in even the most progressive of instances. She humorously expounded on the embrace of paranoia, reflecting on the pervasive utilization of Paul Ricoeur's "hermeneutic of suspicion," even in the face of political conditions that suggested otherwise.[24] Sedgwick argued that paranoia had essentially become methodological: It embraced gloomy affects, was highly anticipatory of the future, and its boisterous negative critiques allowed for no surprises. In short, a paranoid perspective bestowed answers before the questions were even asked. Why, Sedgwick speculated, did queers repeatedly turn to a paranoid predisposition of the world in the face of social, medical, and political advancement? To her, queers were more than happy to elect the monogamy of paranoia over the polyamory of difference and the realities of medical enrichment. Ultimately Sedgwick questioned whether this "uniquely sanctioned method" really made queer lives better or simply provided ready-made conclusions for assorted phenomena. In its place, she called for reparative techniques to cultivate innovative and subversive meaning-making practices that would foster productive strategies for navigating convoluted situations.

Paranoid and reparative reading strategies are not necessarily dichotomous and scholars, including Sedgwick herself, have intimated that anxiety might actually underlie each. Just as apocalyptic discourse can strongly imply longing for utopia, both paranoid sensibilities and reparative desires can stem from the unpleasantries of everyday life, each cruising unrealized dreams in the face of ideological stasis or queer ambivalence about the nature of progress. And, to be sure, paranoia envelops many management frameworks related to both HIV and diabetes because there is no guarantee that ritual care will necessarily prolong one's life. Indeed, Sedgwick speculated on the bleak future of an HIV-positive friend in a segment of the paranoia essay that focuses explicitly on reparative tendencies.[25] Paranoia persists in HIV vernacular, being a recurrent referent in everything from disputes about queer hook-up apps to the anxieties expressed over pre-exposure prophylaxis (PrEP), which has shown to be resoundingly effective in preventing HIV transmission when adherence is maintained.[26] If reparative critiques were underscored by "weak theories" that privileged localize knowledges, AIDS discourse circles back to universal predispositions that centralize paranoia and trauma. The dialectical pairing of apocalypse and utopia, and that of paranoid and reparative, linger in the queer corpus, even if subtly, when HIV is the object of study. Recent developments in queer theory, however, have moved in the direction of precarity and the chronic suffering of populations at the hands of state agencies and capitalist orders. It is not so much that HIV need be fatal, but without proper access to care and modern medicine, perilous circumstances leave people at risk. The analogy to diabetes becomes even more pronounced when this figurative turn is made.

Precarity is a new key word in the critical queer lexicon, emerging concurrently in activist and academic contexts. The concept has been articulated to phenomena as disparate as terrorism and the emergent creative class, although the term was not even listed in some English dictionaries just a few years ago.[27] Scholars engaging the idea of precarity seek to unmask operations of power that exploit vulnerable communities and advocate for ethical imperatives to counteract irreparable harm. In Judith Butler's words, precarity designates "politically induced conditions in which certain populations suffer from failing social and economic networks of support and become differentially exposed to injury, violence, and death."[28] Butler contends that precarity is performatively crafted; only those who are able to reiterate sanctioned cultural norms will be recognized as human to those in power. Without such recognition, no agency is afforded to marginalized people, and the capacity to be undone by oppressive regimes is actualized. The reverberations of apocalypse/utopia and paranoia/reparative resonate in precarity even as this work rarely engages HIV/AIDS, instead finding footing in global economic and labor crises. Nonetheless, the frequent mentions of inaccessible health care in the literature comport well with critical studies of medicine that articulate those at risk of dying from HIV infection and the politics of well-being.

The volatility of HIV/AIDS has gradually morphed in precarity literatures, either rendered to the annals of history or taking on more insipid forms.[29] This progression is noteworthy considering that the affective turn in queer studies directly conjoined paranoia to precarity; the former is built on a foundation of panic and loss that directly informed the latter.[30] AIDS materializes as a study in memory or in the form of a cautionary tale about the perils of poor policy decisions, deficient medical care, and the efforts to garner recognition of non-normative kinships. Butler writes:

> It is worth remembering that one of the main questions that queer theory posed in light of the AIDS crisis was this: How does one live with the notion that one's love is not considered love, and one's loss is not considered loss? How does one live an unrecognizable life? If what and how you love is already a kind of nothing or non-existence, how can you possibly explain the loss of this non-thing, and how would it ever become publicly grievable? Something similar happens when the loss or disappearance of whole populations becomes unmentionable or when the law itself prohibits an investigation of those who committed such atrocities.[31]

I detail the evolution of AIDS rhetoric from apocalyptic to paranoid to precarious not to trivialize the import of such scholarship, which remains vital in a world where rates of HIV transmission remain startlingly high. Nor do I wish to diminish the harsh realities that confront those who are seropositive. Rather, I hope to have established the force of impermanence and foundational relentlessness that continues to lurk beneath the rhetorical composition of HIV. There persists in the above examples an emphasis on the potential for misrecognition, grieving, loss, and disappearance. While activists have successfully incorporated vital world-making practices to redefine safer sex and alleviate stigma, the signifiers associated with HIV continue to lend gravitas to notions of instability and death. Alongside HIV's dire history, diabetes would appear to be a readily controllable condition.

The connotations of consumer capitalism and labor undergirding theories of precarity draw attention to the perils of people attempting to manage conditions in the face of a ravenous for-profit healthcare system. The care of the self is tiresome and is especially confounding when attempted without medical insurance or access to health care. The laborious conditions of daily life suggest not the trauma of apocalyptic discourse, but the dilapidation of the self in everyday life, what Berlant has described elsewhere as a "slow death."[32] Berlant contends that living with HIV is now constituted by an ellipsis, a symbol that suggests both an absence and a bridging device, states of being that have ushered in new subjectivities and normativities related to well-being. How might these refurbished norms and power differentials inform comparisons to diabetes? If scholars are correct in noting that precarious subjects necessitate an Other, the pairing of diabetes and HIV indicates not only an oppositional comparison but one that might also be congruently productive.[33] In most populist literature about precarity, that projected antagonist is the economic 1 percent. In the analogy between HIV and diabetes, it appears to be the lazy diabetic who does little to manage the disease, securing those with HIV in a precarious position and those with diabetes in one that is decrepitly still.

"HIV Is the New Diabetes"

The inspiration for this chapter comes from a pithy remark made by a character on the television program *Nip/Tuck*, who expressed her feelings about being HIV-positive by exclaiming, "HIV is the new diabetes."[34] That this dialogue is embedded in a quasi-medical program known for its whimsy, hyperbole, and cynical critique of America's obsession with aesthetics should not distract from the reality that the analogy is now conventional in the public sphere. Bridging aspects of

HIV and diabetes is routine both in medical vernacular and in internet comment sections, appearing in academic journals, news reports, and scattered throughout popular culture. The connection between the two surfaces in vastly divergent contexts, ranging from debates over immigration policy and HIV status to the morality of bareback porn.[35] Typically, these comparisons are made casually, as when Marie Browne of the Straight and Narrow Medical Day Care noted, "I think the (US government) looks at HIV like diabetes."[36] The parallels are not entirely unwarranted from a medical perspective, as ongoing studies are finding unusual links between the conditions. Some HIV medications have been suspected of initiating type 2 diabetes by killing islet cells, and some drugs spark weight gain, inevitably leading to increased incidences of diabetes. The two diseases also share some consequences if left untreated. Each can lead to the deterioration of the retina and to kidney damage and can cause peripheral neuropathy. Comparisons between the two diseases in medicine are frequent, as more studies are examining the concurrent complications of HIV and diabetes in the United States and abroad.[37] My own endocrinologist has told me that she participates in meetings about the commonalities between HIV and diabetes.

I am not invested here in affirming or negating the viability of the analogy in all instances. In a Foucauldian sense, this discourse is neither wholly regulatory nor entirely liberating. Rather, this portion of the analysis is concerned with the uptake of the analogy to explore the anxieties that surface when diabetes is employed to impart agency to people who are HIV-positive. Those who dismiss the analogy believe management is exclusive to conditions like diabetes, but usually in ways that misunderstand the consequences of glucose irregularities. Even those who embrace the analogy and welcome the reparative potential of the affiliation can oversimplify the ease of diabetes care. I locate fragments of this discourse to discern how the analogy circulates among publics invested in HIV awareness. Those most protective of HIV's unique status stress visions of injurious subjects and paranoid predispositions about medicine, politics, and technology. There is no singular text that best illuminates the ongoing relationship between HIV and diabetes. As such, following the work of scholars such as Bonnie Dow, I take it as a necessity to understand texts and contexts, in this specific case study, as "created, not discovered."[38]

More often than not, people uncomfortable with the association expel outright the analogy between HIV and diabetes. Critics reject the intricacies of analogical reasoning and posit a one-to-one relationship between the conditions that inevitably assumes incommensurability. This tension has been long in the making, preceding technological advancements for both HIV and diabetes. Writing for the HIV resource *The Body* in 1999, Dennis Rhodes contended, "My problem is we've dampened our rage and replaced it with complacency. A lot of people with HIV smoke and drink like there's no tomorrow. And I keep hearing this absurd analogy between HIV disease and diabetes. Excuse me, but you can take my HIV back—I'll take my chances with diabetes."[39] That same year contributors to a journal dedicated to HIV/AIDS and the law wondered if the Americans with Disabilities Act would still protect people who are HIV-positive if they were recognized like those with diabetes.[40] Almost a decade later Clint Walters, the founder of Health Initiatives, rejected the analogy, believing that HIV was more dire than diabetes: "We have the facts and yet we are still missing the message. Don't buy into the myth that HIV is like diabetes. There is nothing manageable when dealing with an uncertain future, side effects from medication and, to top it all off, rejection based purely on your positive status. An HIV diagnosis can rip through your core and make you question everything."[41] AIDS activist Jeff Getty told the Associated Press, "People are thinking, 'Oh I'll just take a pill a day until I'm an old man and everything will be fine.' This is not diabetes. I would love to have diabetes. Compared to HIV, diabetes would be a picnic."[42] An HIV-positive man lamenting advertisements that did not illustrate the side effects of antiretroviral medication exclaimed to *The Oregonian*, "I hear people say it's the new diabetes . . . but it's not."[43] The fears pervading these comments may have been valid at one time, but only if one imagines those with diabetes casually managing the disease and those with HIV at perpetual risk of death.

In each instance, diabetes is visualized as a wholly manageable condition that is seemingly without ramifications. The rendering of diabetes as readily overcome is pervasive in these exchanges, highlighting the extent to which it is imagined as invariable. Complications with insulin, daily struggles with food, the pain associated with injections, and the burdensome costs that accompany care are all elided by an oversimplified discourse of manageability. Disregarding the glut of contingent factors that constitute diabetes gives license to forego the analogy, dispelling innovative possibilities and fortifying staid notions of HIV. The tautology is striking. Those who challenge the analogy trivialize the relationship management has to diabetes, but on the very grounds that they believe management trivializes the effects of HIV.

The preceding remarks comport well with Sedgwick's musings about paranoia being highly anticipatory, affectively negative, and placing much faith in the exposure of analogical failures. The nod to an "uncertain future" Walters mentioned hints at the temporal character of this paranoia, consistently speculating on the struggles that await those who are not vigilant. Chronic conditions are, after all, defined by their relationship to time and the becoming (or disintegration) of the body. And yet this seemingly innocuous statement about the future is telling in its morbid prognostications. There is little room for interpreting the future as anything but bleak, as it is couched in a language that suggests anyone with HIV can predict the (non)surprise of degeneration that awaits. Paranoia's expectant form functions to make visible all mechanisms of oppression and the mendacity of progress narratives that normalize the contours of HIV management.

Although much ink has been spilled attempting to refute analogies to diabetes, these debates are not monolithically one-sided. Where we find apocalyptic projections, we are sure to discover utopic impulses, and where we observe paranoid suspicions, we can always unearth reparative inclinations. The complex interplay of meaning-making by competing factions highlights a still-emerging, frenzied quality to deciphering management rhetorics. The reactionary tone against the analogy was perhaps most powerfully illustrated when columnist Andrew Sullivan published an editorial in the pages of the *Advocate* mocking HIV advocates, whom he saw as exacerbating the effects of HIV, even as people like him lived longer, healthier lives. Sullivan pontificates:

> Far fewer gay men are dying of AIDS anymore. Sometimes local gay papers have no AIDS obits for weeks on end. C'mon, pozzies. You can do better than that! Do you have no sense of social responsibility? Young negative men need to see more of us keeling over in the streets, or they won't be scared enough to avoid a disease that may, in the very distant

future, kill them off. You know, like any other number of diseases that might. They may even stop believing that this is a huge, escalating crisis, threatening to wipe out homosexuality on this planet. What are those happy, HIV-positive men thinking of? Die, damn it.[44]

Sullivan attests that HIV transformed his life, making him a better writer, a healthier person, and a more sexually and spiritually activated gay man. Even as he acknowledges the effects of HIV on some people, he foretells a bright future:

> I'd even be prepared to stop taking my meds if that would help. The trouble is, like many other people with HIV, I did that three years ago. My CD4 count remained virtually unchanged, and only recently have I had to go back on meds. Five pills once a day. No side effects to speak of. I know that others go through far worse, and I don't mean to minimize their trials. But the bottom line is that HIV is fast becoming another diabetes.

Unlike those who dismissed the relation between diabetes and HIV on the grounds that the analogy oversimplified life with HIV, here Sullivan embraces the homology for that very reason. Despite his divergent appropriation of the condition, and his more reparative positioning of HIV, Sullivan shares with the aforementioned critics an oversimplification of life with diabetes. He subscribes to scripts that foster the imagined benefits of "merely" having diabetes and that belief, paradoxically, buttresses notions of diabetes in ways similar to his detractors. It is a theme he would return to when defending the PrEP medication Truvada.[45]

Readers and bloggers retorted that Sullivan was downplaying the negative attributes of living with HIV and accused him of being unaware of the privileged position he occupied. One reader snapped back, using Sullivan's words against him: "Sullivan claims no side effects, but what about the diarrhea, exhaustion, regular doctor visits, and other nuisances that he admits to on his blog? What about the unending worry about infections and the higher incidence of disease among HIV-positive folks? This is no diabetes."[46] Thomas Gegeny, executive director of the Center for AIDS Information and Advocacy, countered, "Extolling the newly dubbed descriptions of HIV as 'another diabetes' (i.e., a chronic, manageable condition) is appealing, but what about the myriad health problems faced by people with HIV, whether on or off medicine?"[47] Rebuking Sullivan, one blogger wrote, "HIV medications don't work for everyone; I know this first-hand: my virus is resistant or intolerant to most of them. Unlike diabetes, HIV is associated with damning social stigma and pozzies bear the burden of becoming a carrier of a deadly virus."[48] Of the many letters and blog posts written against Sullivan's position, I could find only one that condemns him for potentially misrepresenting diabetes.[49]

Skeptics occasionally reconstruct the rhetorical scaffolding that frames the analogy to ensure diabetes remains static compared with the dynamic nature of HIV. Even in cases where it would appear a reparative approach is being taken up, the comparison is manipulated to guide an interpretation of HIV's inconstancy. Such was the case when John-Manuel Andriote published an editorial on the *Huffington Post* titled, "HIV Is 'Like Diabetes'? Let's Stop Kidding Ourselves." After carefully detailing the challenges and complications confronting people with diabetes, Andriote refocused his attention from management to cure. It's worth quoting him at length to illustrate fully this sleight of hand and the wounded attachment he crafts:

> We need to banish the notion that HIV infection today is 'like diabetes,' in spite of their similarities. Consider:
>
> Both are transmitted through intimate behavior, one through sex, and the other, frequently, through family habits passed down over generations. Both diseases are alike in that they are best avoided and challenging to manage. They both cost a great deal of money for medications, medical specialists, and lab work. Certainly, HIV and diabetes each could destroy your health and likely kill you if they aren't properly managed. As for people with type-two diabetes seeking to manage their illness, a healthy diet and exercise strengthen an HIV-positive person's ability to handle the daily impact of toxic chemotherapies; the hassle of medical appointments and blood work every few months; the discipline of taking pills every day, and dealing with their physical side effects; and the emotional, financial, and psychological tolls of having a financially and socially expensive medical condition.
>
> But beyond this, and in spite of the obvious differences between a viral disease and a metabolic one, the most striking difference between having

HIV and type-two diabetes today is this: There's not even a remote chance that changing my diet or exercise habits can cure what I have.

If only.[50]

Andriote handcuffs himself to the precarity of illness, stifling a nuanced and original exposition with oversimplification and shaming in the space of a few words. Even in the face of extensive similarities, he positions diabetes as easily eliminated by alterations in diet or physical activity.

In fairness, the anxiety expressed by many of the aforementioned activists and writers is not fabricated out of thin air; there is strong precedent for distrusting that HIV is on the brink of being cured. People with HIV continue to be undone by the devastating effects of stigma, medical complications, and economic hardship. The concern expressed by people assailing the analogy exhibits a distrust of stability and comfort because advocates want people to remain vigilant against HIV's dangers.[51] In this way, they are justified in dramatizing the uncertainty that confronts many people with HIV. Invocations of management potentially occlude the quotidian struggles faced by people who do not have access to health care, medicine, and social support services. We should not forget that HIV, like diabetes, is increasingly a problem experienced by the poor. And, as Berlant reminds us, those on the lowest rung of the socioeconomic spectrum are not quick to embrace additional struggles or stigmas.[52] Even those who have resources grapple with the daily contours of chronic conditions that dilapidate their worlds at a glacial pace. These commonalities might potentially create kinship among diabetes and HIV, but the rhetoric often signals a move toward estrangement and not conviviality.

Rather than accept these depictions of the analogy, we might productively engage the germane qualities of HIV and diabetes that offer insight into management rhetorics. Prevalent notions of choice, for instance, undergird many of the paranoid proclivities outlined above. In the aforementioned examples, fault for everything from health to interpretive choices is placed in the hands of individuals. Rhodes berated people with HIV who continued to smoke and drink without restraint. Walters implored his readers not to "buy into the myth" that HIV is like diabetes. Sullivan said he would *willingly* go off his meds to prove his point. And at every turn there was a suggestion that people were purposefully careless because they could simply take pills to continue living. The trope of choice across these narratives maintains a focus on individual bodies, rather than systemic features that might alter the face of care. The arguments forwarded by both proponents and opponents of the analogy assume that others are easily interpellated by management discourses at every turn. Choice reifies management, giving continual, if not unintentional, power to discipline bodies. To echo Foucault, management is a trap.

The amplification of individualism by those resistant to the analogy also hints at an apprehension about the evolving role of AIDS in activist politics and queer communities. HIV activism has proven most effective when it focuses not simply on personal fortitude, but on political systems complicit in the deaths of people most marginalized by economic greed and medical neglect. A refrain such as "HIV is the new diabetes" focuses on no such things. The expression can be interpreted as conceptually aesthetic in nature—it is literally based on the fashion metaphor "X is the new black." Systems are erased completely in this catchphrase, putting pressure on individuals to stay well without consideration of the resources necessary to cultivate the imagined norms of health. Finally, and this cannot be overstated enough, diabetes is an unusual anchor for this position. People with diabetes, like people with HIV, struggle with the subjugation of normativities, uncertain futures, and the stigma brought about by able-bodied publics that focus on the coterminous relationship among excess, neglect, and moral failing. To think through the potential of the analogy, I will next invert the pairing, attempting to discern what HIV might tell us about diabetes not as rhetorically sedentary, but as vivaciously contingent.

"Maybe Diabetes Is the New HIV?"

I delivered a version of this book's introduction at an invited talk, one in which the analogy was mentioned only in passing, and an audience member who was struck by its inclusion said to me, "maybe diabetes is the new HIV?" As a scholar who had studied HIV/AIDS for many years, I scoffed at the suggestion. To my mind the legacy of AIDS was rooted in Treichler's crisis of signification, stigmatized bodies, overcoming shame, marginalized populations, bustling movements, and economic struggles to afford treatment. And yet, the more I ran through that list in my mind, the more the analogy resonated. Although the development of each disease's etiology has noteworthy differences, the two share similarities in this particular historical moment that are equally enlightening. Scholarship on analogies tells us that some shared characteristics among the objects being appraised must be plausible to an audience for the juxtaposition to be successful.[53] These "proposals of resemblance," S. Scott Graham observes, leave open the possibility of communicators accepting or rejecting an analogy in any given situation.[54] Of course, the integrity of any analogy is rhetorically constructed, being judged by publics that are primed to assess contrasts in culturally specific ways. The sanctioning of particular articulations as probable is not a transparent process, but one inflected by communal values, refined contexts, and the predispositions of the audience assessing the likenesses. If we can shift our perspectives ever so slightly to entertain the feasibility that "diabetes is the new HIV," then significant parallels emerge among the conditions.

The previous segment of this chapter illustrated that people engaging the analogy almost always fashion HIV as a dexterous infection and diabetes as an ailment that is functionally stable. It does not matter if one searches the internet for the words "HIV and diabetes" or "diabetes and HIV," the outcome remains the same—HIV is afforded protean qualities and diabetes is figured as a steady, unchangeable point of comparison. Despite the reliability of these search engine results, a subtle conversion has occurred in public debates that enlist the analogy. The relationship among the two has moved from being ludicrous to plausible to, most recently, inverted. HIV is now being touted as the more manageable disease, and examples of this transposition are materializing rapidly. An analogy can take sharp turns in meaning because its parts are not stable mechanisms; rather, they spark infinite interpretive results when weighed by different actors. Take for example the candidacy of Democrat Bob Poe, who announced he was running for Congress in 2016. The analogy became a fixture of his campaign rhetoric.[55] Poe has been HIV-positive since the late 1990s and proclaimed that, "We've got to rip the mask off this thing and begin talking about it in a sensible way . . . [HIV] is a chronic condition that is more easily treated than diabetes."[56] Interestingly, in some of the media narratives focusing on Poe where the analogy is not explicitly stated, readers in comment sections have debated its appropriateness.[57]

Perhaps most famously, Dr. Max Pemberton invoked the analogy in an editorial published in *The Spectator* where he contended that HIV was the easier disease to manage.[58] Pemberton, who was trained as a physician at the height of the AIDS crisis, reflected on the progress that has transformed the life expectancies of people living with HIV. The doctor relayed that he had not witnessed a single death due to complications from HIV in several years, even including among high-risk groups such as sex workers. Pointing to revolutions in AIDS research, Pemberton testified that the "medical profession now considers HIV a chronic disease; it's regarded in public health terms in the same category as, for example, type 2 diabetes. As a doctor I can tell you that, medically speaking, I'd rather have HIV than diabetes." Pemberton mentioned the various complications that often result from diabetes, such as cardiovascular disease, the need for dialysis, nerve damage, and the loss of sight. He acknowledged that stigmatizing social attitudes toward people with HIV have not kept pace with medical advancements. Still, longevity rates among people with diabetes are about a decade shorter than that of the average person, whereas life projections for people with HIV are now equal to those who are seronegative.[59]

To be sure, Pemberton's response could be interpreted as a paranoid reading of life with diabetes. Giving attention to death, blindness, amputations, and heart attacks does not project an optimistic take on an already lurid condition. Yet the performative interruption of reiterating diabetes as stable in this dialectical pairing might accomplish much in replotting one of the largest misperceptions people have about the condition—that it takes little effort to control. Sedgwick reminds us that "reparative practices are additive and accretive," altering cultural conditions, sometimes at a seemingly glacial pace. A reparative approach might be anxiety-driven, but "its fear, a realistic one, is the culture surrounding it is inadequate or inimical to its nurture; it wants to assemble and confer plentitude on an object that will then have resources to offer to an inchoate self."[60] As the chronic features of diabetes and HIV grow more noticeable, we must continue to mine the prospects inherent in their composition, especially those that engender worthwhile conversations about public health and collective action. Rather than relegating diabetes as a sedentary condition, this affinity would privilege a destabilization of significations, scrutinize the stratification of illness, and reveal how bodies materialize as "impure." In what follows, I look to rhetorical resemblances that are reparative in their inclination, troubling habitual iterations of diabetes. The analogy can unsettle unreflective claims about management, detailing the instability, if not precariousness, that underwrites deliberation about diabetes. I look to three nodal points: the shaming tendencies that are ubiquitous in public dialogue about each disease, heedless calls for abstaining that function to stigmatize those living with chronic illness, and the positionality of raced bodies in the constitution of diabetes and HIV.

The Specter of Shame

The cultural schemas of diabetes and HIV hold noteworthy parallels that rest outside the reductive logics of management, but those commonalities are often given short shrift in public appraisals of the analogy. Take, for example, the myriad ways shame is used to discipline people whose eating habits or sexual proclivities are judged as aberrant, even when they are practices that are otherwise socially encouraged and commonly performed. Shame has stunted collective action and frustrated structural changes and in the process marginalized and stigmatized those most in need of assistance. This was clearly the case with HIV/AIDS, where political and personal shame inhibited responses to the crisis, locating arduous struggles in the private sphere, denying the public character of the epidemic and the resources needed to keep people alive. President Ronald Reagan's refusal to say "AIDS" in public for six full years after the initial outbreak, activist efforts to bring people out of the closet to curtail infection rates, and the aversion to safer-sex education all reflected, albeit in vastly divergent manners, the ways shame animated HIV's havoc. As late as spring 2016, I was privy to a conversation in which someone, who is too young to remember the appalling indifference and hostility directed at people with HIV/AIDS at the dawn of the epidemic, off-handedly commented that she knew someone who contracted HIV "through no fault of her own." The refrain parrots some of the most troubling, even if well-intentioned, rhetoric of the 1980s and 1990s, indicating the presence of a person or group that shoulders the weight of their serostatus while others are stratified as helpless in the face of unforeseen circumstances. A fleeting thought makes explicit the challenges that continue to confront people who are HIV-positive decades after HIV's arrival. This ceaselessly creeping shame has motivated some queer counter-publics to mobilize shame as a retort to traditional invocations of LGBT pride, which often have the consequence of reiterating normative structures that privilege some queers and deprecate others.[61] There is little room here to detail the ways shame has instigated inspired critiques of political movements or how such rhetorics are built on a foundation that could be read as simultaneously paranoid and reparative. Suffice to say that people with HIV have long been accused of initiating their own demise through their sexual prowess or reckless obsessions. In the analogy to diabetes, a likeminded trope is forged with those who could have prevented their ailments by eating healthier or implementing more vigorous exercise regimens.

Shame crafts a blunt hierarchy of accountability in rhetorics about diabetes and HIV, with sharp distinctions being made between those who are regarded as innocent bystanders of disease and those who were complicit in their own diagnosis. Just as the acquaintance above relayed knowledge of a person who seroconverted in a situation not of their own making, people with type 1 diabetes are routinely cast as sympathetic victims who are randomly affected by an environmental trigger. Such people were generally diagnosed as children and their fate is rightfully construed as a product of circumstance and not behavior. Like hemophiliacs and those who received HIV through blood transfusions, or wives and girlfriends who were infected because of their partners' alleged promiscuity, people with type 1 diabetes are often situated as "innocent victims" of a predatory disease who stand in contradistinction to those guilty of welcoming disease. Of course, I am not suggesting we should lodge more guilt in the direction of people with type 1 diabetes. Rather, I offer caution about the unbridled stigmatization of people with type 2 diabetes, not only because caustic accusations are injurious and demoralizing but also because such discourse inevitably circles back to people with type 1 diabetes in adulthood. The schism between deserving recipients and innocent victims was rarely useful in AIDS histories, perpetuating stigma and pain in communities already grappling with the stress of a brutal and incurable constellation of ailments. Unfortunately, in discussions of diabetes the individuation of disease is rehearsed time and again, usually at the expense of structural changes that would help save lives.

Even within diabetes communities accusatory rhetorics circulate unabashedly and with great bravado. So strong is the division among people with type 1 and type 2 diabetes that many in the former group have called for a new name to make their condition distinct from the other. A petition on change.org has collected almost 10,000 signatures calling for a name change for type 1 diabetes. Following the publication of an essay on the website *DiabetesHealth.com* asserting that people with type 1 diabetes could learn important lessons from those with type 2, message boards erupted. Some in the media went as far as proclaiming a "civil war" among the groups.[62] One reader turned to management imagery, writing angrily:

> Type 1 DM [diabetes mellitus] and Type 2 are completely different diseases with different etiologies. I have had Type 1 for 28 years now and am so tired of people assuming I am lazy and eat horribly. I did nothing to give myself this disease. If my beloved endocrinologist told me "Ya' know, if you eat a bit better and lost about 40 pounds, your diabetes would likely go away," I would be a perfect size 6 in no time flat. Type 2s have it easy.

Whereas people with type 1 diabetes are situated as motivated and health-oriented despite their diagnosis, those with type 2 are imagined as simultaneously overindulgent and static, certainly without the motivation to overcome their desires. The person making the above claim demonstrates her responsible disposition, detailing an intimate relationship with a medical specialist and claiming the wherewithal to make choices that would vanquish diabetes. Another reader angrily contended, "I have been type 1 for 46 years (I'm 50), and I have yet to meet a type 2 who is, and has always been a 'health-concious [sic] eater.'" Anecdotal evidence is incorporated as a technique of surveillance by the respondent, imparting not medical knowledge but moral rebuke. In this reader's mind, people with type 2 diabetes brought the disease upon themselves because they did not have the fortitude to manage their gluttony. The paradox is stunning when we consider the idle connotations of the disease: Even as diabetes is seen as a product of laziness and neglect, the degree of excess implied is bountiful. In the above scenario, people with type 2 diabetes can master their condition (indeed, make it disappear) if only they exert an unspecified but seemingly prudent amount of effort. If we replace HIV with type 1 diabetes in this example, it would comport fluidly with detractors of the analogy who profess the ease of management and the dire nature of their troubles. Tellingly, the retort mirrors the spirit of Andriote's claims about HIV and diabetes noted earlier in this chapter. The apocalyptic sensibility, the paranoid tone, and the precarious subject position converge to cast those with type 2 as self-made social outliers.

The normativities lurking in suppositions about diabetes and HIV fortify stigma by positing a body that actively invited decline, giving way to passions it cannot fully rein in. Failure to maintain health is regarded as an individual choice that is stripped of context, nuance, and data that might challenge conjectural suppositions. Responding to the exchanges among people with types 1 and 2 diabetes, one commentator on *Diabetesdaily.com* harshly proclaimed that type 2 was the "wuss version" of the disease. She went on to say, in all caps, "NO TYPE 2 COULD EVER DO WHAT I HAVE DONE FOR THE PAST 28 YEARS . . . IT IS NOT THE SAME. NOT EVEN CLOSE. HOW DARE YOU."[63] The reader chides an imagined persona, one whose will is void of motivation and whose attempts at shared identification with type 1 diabetes are read as patently offensive. There is no effort at dialogue in such retorts, only the intention to rebuff others regardless of circumstance. Stigma is reproduced by the reader, contributing to an atmosphere that stymies any trace of identification, much less strategies for wellness. It is worth repeating that the blame people with type 2 diabetes experience inspires so much guilt that it customarily incites chronic depression. Importantly, so does living with HIV, whose materialization is consistently posited as retrospectively preventable. The constant reminders that choice summoned disease often has the effect of making people despondent. As River Solomon, an author with type 2 diabetes, wrote in the *New York Times*, "A lifetime of dieting, a lifetime of being told my body is wrong, takes its toll, and I can't help conflating the messages that I am better off starved than fat. Maybe if I could let go of the shame, or more important, if the media, doctors, friends, family could stop shaming me, managing my diabetes wouldn't be this roulette wheel of self-torture."[64]

Cvetkovich reminds us that depression is a public feeling not easily reduced to oversimplified scripts of personal sovereignty.[65] The sedentary connotations that mark diabetes, in this case type 2 diabetes, mask dangerous undercurrents of liberal individualism that do not appropriately address the more onerous aspects of chronic disease.

A Subject Free of Desire

The knee-jerk reaction to shame people with diabetes and reaffirm a guilty subject in need of behavior modification suggests migration toward a scapegoat, one whose body must be purified but without consideration of the messy entanglements that constitute the sociality of this chronic condition. Although abstinence may seem like an unusual corollary to derive from the analogy to HIV, one only need swap "abstinence" with "control" to see the relay from one to the other. There were fewer moves as sundry and diabolical in HIV's history than calls for abstinence, a removal of the self from the likelihood of contamination, literally a subject who should not desire. The historical consistency of calling on people to abstain from sex is striking. In May 1987, the Moral Majority's Newspaper the *Liberty Report* preached that gay men should stop having sex to prevent AIDS from destroying the American family. The paper admonished readers: "As AIDS prevention becomes the key element in this national health crisis, one topic not addressed in the early stages of the epidemic is beginning to be heard—that abstinence is the best policy . . . Morality, for several alarming reasons, has once again become vogue."[66] Humankind will be cleansed only when non-institutionally sanctioned sex is sacrificed, giving way to a moral utopia that rewards compliance. Echoes of this jeremiad have persisted over the decades, and calls for abstinence from anti-gay factions are equally fashionable today. As late as June 2016, conservative news sites lambasted President Obama for not advising gay men to stop having sex to avoid HIV's transmission.[67] Of course, abstinence has never been a particularly effective strategy for eradicating HIV. Indeed, reputable studies from sources that range from the *Lancet* to the United Nations have found that the surest way to wipe out HIV would be to make gay sex legal worldwide.[68] Public health officials and HIV activists have long insisted that if the stigma of HIV were removed and the paranoia associated with sexuality displaced, then spaces could be opened for productive conversations about sex and prevention. Those who want to simply wish away the complicated social character of HIV are ill informed and their chaste proposals are often underwritten by misogynistic and homophobic scripts that highlight personal responsibility and virtuous citizenship. In many corners of the United States, teens and young adults continue to be put at risk by abstinence-only education programs and ineffective virginity pledges, which repeatedly result in higher rates of pregnancy and disease transmission.[69] These tendencies are hardly isolated to the far Right. Organizations such as the AIDS Healthcare Foundation, one of the largest AIDS providers in the country, continues to deny the use of PrEP as a public health tool, using caustic and morally damning rhetoric to persuade gay men that technologies proven to enact safer sex are not working.

Present-day calls for people with type 2 diabetes to simply eat less and exercise more mirror these utopic and unrealistic pleas for abstinence. Just as telling a person not to have sex masks the social and relational nature of sex and sexuality, so too does castigating a person for eating fail to consider opportunities for contemplating the pleasures associated with consumption, the convivial joy of sharing meals, and the ways that food, like sex, is a reflection of cultural structures of desire. In place of these cliché criticisms, attention should be given to quotidian practices that account for the myriad tendencies of people to consume that rest outside notions of liberal individualism and choice. Food and sex are two of the foundational needs of Maslow's hierarchy, yet those eager to shame suggest that if we eradicate these base necessities then self-actualization might magically be achieved. Rather than allege that people with diabetes are too laissez-faire in their self-management, we might consider which choices are provided across the socioeconomic spectrum and how people are enabled (or not) to render decisions.[70]

Returning briefly to the "civil war" between people with types 1 and 2 diabetes crystallizes the degree to which abstinence is often interwoven into debates about care, even if indirectly. In June 2015, CrossFit CEO Greg Glassman tweeted an image of a bottle of Coca-Cola that read "Open Diabetes." Underneath the image were the words, "Make sure you pour some out for your dead homies" and the hashtag #Sugarkills. The message was clear: Soda consumption is tantamount to grave digging.

Buying into expensive exercise programs, on the other hand, is an act of salvation. The word "homies" is awkwardly racialized, especially in light of the fact that CrossFit clientele tend to be upper-middle-class whites.[71] The next day singer and actor Nick Jonas, who lives with type 1 diabetes, tweeted back, "This is not cool. Please know and understand the difference between type one and type [two] diabetes before making ignorant comments." Social media users reacted quickly, pointing out that Jonas's remarks, while well intentioned, also reinforced a stratification of culpability. Jonas quickly retooled his tweet to read, "Ignorant comments. Sensitivity to all diseases, and proper education on the cause and day to day battle is important." There is no shortage of links made between diabetes and consumption in Western culture, but even subtle messages of restraint and shame are omnipresent. To offer one more example: In April 2016, a Florida man complained after a Starbucks barista wrote "Diabetes here I come" on his drink receipt. The man has two sisters who have type 1 diabetes and he found the note distasteful, being little more than a mechanism to surveil and humiliate unsuspecting patrons. It would seem people with (and in this case without) diabetes must abstain lest they be mocked by total strangers and made to feel as though they were engaging in inappropriate behavior. This man's instinct that such messages have a negative impact on people with diabetes is not mistaken. Informal surveys have found that upwards of 72 percent of people believe that the stigma associated with the disease comes from a "failure of personal responsibility" above all other factors.[72]

Self-aggrandizing moralizers who demand ever more control of libidinous urges are a recurrent presence in the histories of both diabetes and HIV. In noting these parallels, however, I am not attempting to create a one-to-one analogical correspondence among the ways these disciplinary tendencies are executed. Perelman's contention that analogies reflect degrees of proportionality provides an important caveat, one that tempers the malleability of the analogy and calls attention to situated reasoning. Excessive eating, for example, is not likely to materialize as the new "unsafe sex" any time soon. Then again, in an era of PrEP use, what was once considered unsafe sex is now under definitional scrutiny. New technologies are easing the need for unending self-surveillance and drastically interrupting the ways both these medical phenomena are put into discourse, even as factions suspicious of uninhibited inclinations toward food or sex continue to urge unending self-restraint. The fear of a desirous subject whose body is out of bounds is certainly nothing new. Sontag noted the cultural parallels between sexual deviancy, excessiveness, and overindulgence when she wrote *AIDS and Its Metaphors* years ago.[73] Kathleen LeBesco has observed a similar theme, arguing that stigma is often reproduced on the bodies of people who are accused of insatiable lust, whether in relation to sex or food.[74] When articulated to a racialized body, these social trepidations become even more hyperbolic, disciplinary, and wrought with moral panic.

Racial Classifications and the Typification of Diabetes

Finally, the long tradition of conjoining disease to demands for sacrifice, personal responsibility, and culturally sanctioned norms raises questions about those people most likely to endure surveillance from disapproving critics. HIV's legacy demonstrates that potent erasures and undue condemnation are fixtures of medical practices, public policy, and media coverage. People of color have been the object of discipline when their experiences do not comport to universal notions of treatment or sensationalized media scripts. The selective attention offered to communities of color continues to exacerbate present-day medical quandaries, especially diabetes diagnoses among Native Americans and African Americans, the latter of whom have long suffered disproportionate rates of HIV diagnosis for a host of political and cultural reasons. Of course, one need not engage the similarities between diabetes and HIV to recognize the role that race has played in both the history and discursive materialization of disease. That has been well established. However, recent invocations of the analogy point to the incongruent burdens faced by people of color and the caustic rhetoric that seeks to regulate their bodies.[75]

Momentarily returning to Andrew Sullivan's writings reveals how rhetorics of management and race linger in the analogy between diabetes and HIV. In a 1996 *New York Times Magazine* article titled "When Plagues End," Sullivan famously trumpeted that we were finally in the "twilight of an epidemic."[76] At the time, Sullivan argued that HIV no longer promised death, but "merely signifies illness." Such proclamations were made just as HIV rates among minorities and the poor were rapidly expanding. People were able to live longer and healthier lives, but only if they had the means necessary to stay well. Phillip Brian Harper, C. Riley Snorton, and Cathy Cohen have each maintained that racist and nationalistic impulses ground Sullivan's account, as most of his analysis excluded considerations of racial minorities.[77] As Snorton notes, Sullivan's disavowal is "informed by an ignorance of the impact of AIDS on blacks, Latinos, poor people, and drug users, all routinely underreported in the news coverage of HIV/AIDS."[78] Racial minorities have long confronted institutional and media neglect and, as Kevin Mumford has carefully documented, African American activists were largely left to their own devices when it came to gathering resources and spreading information about AIDS when it emerged as a threat.[79]

Sullivan's use of the analogy discussed earlier in this chapter is not necessarily mistaken, but it does raise important questions about the bodies being imagined in accounts drawing on the comparison. As with his *When Plague Ends* essay, the headway made in medicine does not necessarily translate to strides made among actual people. And when progress is made by some and not others, there is a tendency to blame those most affected by disease for their condition. Cathy Cohen cautions against these stunting rhetorics of blame and personal responsibility that disingenuously castigate African Americans for rates of HIV infection, and her exhortation can be fluidly extended to diabetes.[80] Cohen singles out Bill Cosby as an especially egregious (if not tragically ironic) user of the trope of "personal responsibility" when lecturing black audiences about HIV. Interestingly, the comic also employed diabetes to underscore a "plague of apathy" theme, telling communities of color they must make better choices to live higher quality lives.[81] He told one audience: "It becomes a term of apathy because people say my father had it, my aunt had it. People then ask you, 'What your mother die of?' 'Diabetes.' 'Grandmother?' 'Diabetes.' These things don't have to happen if you make the correct choice." Racial minorities are metonymically reduced to disease, represented as holding the very key to success if only they were not fettered by their poor decision making. This synopsis overlooks a range of contributing factors that complicate systemic considerations of ailments. If we looked, not at individual bodies but at locations that reported high rates of diabetes, for example, a fuller account of how diabetes manifests might be recognized. In places such as New York,

Detroit, and Atlanta, all of which have sizeable communities of color, diabetes rates are highest in those parts of the city that are poor and where services like grocery stores are sometimes not found for miles. Metaphors such as "food deserts" obscure the man-made nature of such locations, depicting a naturalized account of poverty. People are often stuck, but not simply because of individual choices. African Americans constitute less than 13 percent of the population but are 77 percent more likely to develop diabetes than their white counterparts. Structural remedies must engage questions of health care, Medicare and Medicaid support, the ubiquity of fast food in low-income neighborhoods, and attitudes toward consumption. If diabetes is indeed the new HIV, that status is accompanied by social, and not simply medical, analogies.

Unreflective assumptions about race, diabetes, and risk are especially worrisome because they often function to ratify preexisting assumptions about minorities. There is a striking discrepancy in the scientific literature between the risk of inheriting type 1 diabetes and type 2 diabetes among different racial groups. The risk of developing type 1 diabetes is presented as decisively high among white people.[82] Conversely, those at the greatest risk for type 2 diabetes in the United States are Native Americans, African Americans, Latinos, Asian Americans, and finally those classified as white. The fact that those with type 1 diabetes are generally framed as "innocent" and those with type 2 as "guilty" should, at the very least, instigate reflection about predetermined racial frames. Scholars ranging from Troy Duster to Kelly Happe have warned against presupposing genetic risk models are at the root of all medical diagnoses, encouraging a sustained focus on the cultural influences that reinforce problematic assumptions underlying medical determinism.[83] As Duster cautions, there is no magic bullet in genetic research about health disorders connected to racial minorities, but once research is under way, medical nomenclatures can overwhelm scientific lexicons and conventional wisdom alike. Genetic ascriptions of diabetes, for example, often fortify preexisting prejudices about ethnic and racial identities that are not supported by evidence. This is not to say that racial minorities are not at risk for diabetes, it simply means those risks might be more environmental and social than genetically foreordained. Associating the "risk" factors of diabetes with presumptions about work ethic, dependency, and responsibility creates circumstances where the potential for scapegoating becomes frighteningly real. People of color are frequently shunned for everything from "lifestyle choices" (a language that should ring familiar to those invested in the legacy of HIV) to rhetoric suggesting that they do not manage passions (a theme I will return to in chapter 4). The comparison to HIV should stimulate the capacity for contemplating the extent of the analogy's fungibility, not merely staid notions of management.

"The Diabetes Apocalypse Is Upon Us"

The ways HIV rhetorically inflects the analogy to diabetes provides one opportunity for, in Kenneth Burke's terminology, *attitudinizing* novel understandings of the condition. That is, the terms used and excluded in discussions of health and medicine are not merely descriptive but furnish the material for conceptualizing disease anew. The persistent dismissal of the analogy is acceptable only to the extent that one situates diabetes as essentially tranquil. And yet, if we look closely at diabetes, we know that it is a complex and dynamic disease not easily surmised in its origins, manifestations, or complications, just as HIV is not. In detailing the ways diabetes and HIV inform one another, I have not intended to reinforce a static binary nor insist that an inversion of the analogy equivocates discrepancies among the two. Nonetheless, there are subtle ways in which the chronic conditions have influenced one another's public character. Take, for example, the ascendance of the phrase "people with diabetes." As opposed to the more ubiquitous "diabetic," "people with diabetes" pays homage to the influence of AIDS activism in diabetes rhetoric. The emphasis on personhood and the unwillingness to be reduced to disease is increasingly employed in diabetes communities by those attempting to stunt the reproduction of stigma that often accompanies living with the condition. These changes are indebted to the work of both HIV and diabetes activists and those efforts are not easily unknotted.

The analogy to HIV has tended to incite criticism of diabetes as a product of motionless bodies that are slowly languishing away. This attitude obscures the similarities each have as extra-medico texts unconfined to the rationalistic tendencies of modernity. The metaphors for each have not simply been casually health-oriented, but hyperbolically incited as threats to the very fabric of humanity. AIDS, for instance, materialized regularly through metaphors actualizing it as a military threat, a foreign invasion, an earthquake, pollution, the apocalypse, and a plague.[84] Diabetes has likewise been awakened through tropes such as terrorism, floods, death marches, shipwrecks, aggression, and addiction.[85] This manifestation of danger can be found in headlines that proclaim, "City Stalked by Diabetes" and "Diabetes: Don't Let This Chronic Illness Hold You Hostage."[86] The recurring referents of danger, contamination, excess, and boundary crossing point to the resistive force of each disease, highlighting the precarity of human life in the face of apocalyptic fissures. Some of these figures suggest circumstances designed by people and are therefore open to reproach; others are conceived as natural phenomena and ostensibly unstoppable. Although many of the tropes are collective in nature, systemic redress is often elided and shared struggles are relocated to the singularity of disease management typical of Western medicine. Nonetheless, the images also illustrate the common language of threat utilized to assess dilemmas and introduce solutions.

The implications to be gleaned from exploring the relationship between HIV and diabetes should give us pause, especially since conditions such as Alzheimer's are increasingly being linked to diabetes. Attention to stigma heralds a warning about the ways analogies can reiterate patterns of social shaming that negatively affect treatment and care. As mentioned in the previous chapter, the suggestion that Alzheimer's might be caused, in part, by complications from glucose regulation troubles conventional understandings of the disease. The brain produces some insulin and is rich with insulin receptors because the organ requires glucose to function. The connections being made among blood sugar, brain capacity, and in some cases obesity are not entirely surprising, since for years doctors have recorded a decrease in cognitive and mental capacities with elevated glucose levels. Experts hope if glycemic intake can be regulated more closely earlier in life, the development of Alzheimer's might be stalled. It is still too early to know if Alzheimer's will come to be known exclusively as *type 3 diabetes*, but the stigma suggested in the analog between HIV and diabetes should signal cultural, and not simply medical, problems.[87] Knowing that people with type 2 diabetes are blamed for their demise, one must wonder if the same would come to pass for those with Alzheimer's. The current significations attached to Alzheimer's are not as malicious when contemplating origins, but this new placement, should it take hold, could open avenues for executing harsh judgments and imparting people with an agency over a condition that they never controlled. I do not mean to be dismal in the face of medical breakthroughs, only to state that shifting the language from "Alzheimer's disease" to "type 3 diabetes" would come not only with new possibilities for research and perhaps a cure, but also with novel opportunities for disciplining ailing bodies.

As diabetes rates continue to climb, rhetorics actualizing a state of emergency seem to be materializing at an ever-expanding rate. Anxieties that reiterate the impulses of apocalypse, paranoia, and precariousness come easily when confronted with the looming possibility of more lives lost to disease. As the analogy continues to strengthen there will no doubt be a strong tendency to accentuate projections of peril and despair. Articles pronouncing a forthcoming "diabetes apocalypse" in China and Australia, for example, have recently graced internet news reports. Following a 2014 report about diabetes in the *Lancet*, one news source declared that "the diabetes apocalypse is upon us." Still another proclaimed that fear, guilt, anger, and shame were the four horsemen of the diabetes apocalypse. These predictions do little to remedy the ills brought to bear by diabetes, ignoring the reparative prospects of public health, technological advancement, and expanding healthcare options. A charitable read of alarmist rhetoric might find that institutional action could be incited to prevent the escalation of chronic disease rates. Imagining HIV as the new diabetes, or diabetes as the new HIV, need not forecast alarmist rhetorics of demise, just as it need not overstate the case of managing diabetes.

As diabetes continues to become more globally prominent, it will be even more imperative to craft alternatives for putting the condition into discourse, disarticulating its relationship to shame, blame, and the ease of management. What if our discourses emphasized more insidious forms of management that regress from the presuppositions of individual responsibility? What if we gave presence to the pains associated with needle sticks and shots experienced daily by those living with diabetes? How might we save lives if we highlighted the variability of resources and the need for universal health care? How might issues of choice be divorced from diabetes when we consider the trappings of geography, depression, and support? Rather than enforce a discourse of management that renders these complications invisible, as the analogy between HIV and diabetes frequently does for both diseases, new narratives might be construed to activate workable alternatives. New remedies need to be explored, ones that engage the artistry with which people regulate their health and the methods that can be used to offer visibility to their pain. The next chapter looks to a similar instance of cataclysmic rhetoric, but one that is employed to instigate federal resources, not to shame populations. The JDRF's fatal perspective on diabetes has invariably proven to be effective in marshalling such means. Despite the dark premise, their approach is oddly reparative and their voices heard by some of the most powerful political figures in the world.

3

Lethal Premonitions

Fatalism and Advocacy

Most people think of complications as something that happens to older people or after you have had diabetes for a very long time. I am here to tell you that it is just not true. Look around this room, there is no way for you to know how many of these children are already experiencing problems with their kidneys or their eyes, because diabetes is silent. On the outside, we look healthy. On the inside, a war is raging in our bodies, a war we cannot fight alone.
—Caroline Rowley, age eleven, 2001

In July 2006, five years after he first took office, President George W. Bush was confronted with the reality of his first executive veto. Defying threats from the White House, Congress had passed legislation allowing couples who had pursued in vitro fertilization to donate unused embryos, that would otherwise be discarded, to be used in stem cell research. It was a politically isolating experience for the president, who lacked support from both legislative chambers and upwards of 70 percent of the American people. Put in the unusual position of playing defense against a Republican majority, the administration responded by calling a press conference and surrounding Bush with children. The "snowflake" babies, as they were called, were children born from surplus embryos created by in vitro fertilization and given over to couples who were having trouble reproducing. Bush presented the minors as a visual testament to his staunch opposition to embryonic stem cell research, a policy position that would stunt the prospect of curing Alzheimer's, Parkinson's, and diabetes. Bush told the audience of reporters gathered in the East Room of the White House that the kids were not "spare parts," asserting their worth as people and enthymematically suggesting that stem cell research was tantamount to murder. The American people, he declared, "must remember that embryonic stem cells come from human embryos that are destroyed for their cells. Each of these human embryos is a unique human life with inherent dignity and matchless value. We see that value in the children who are with us today." Where the president found dignity and moral purpose, critics assailed his decision as just one more example of the White House's narrowed exaltations about "life." Indeed, after years of support from his conservative allies, Bush found himself at odds with a number of high-profile Republicans that included former First Lady Nancy Reagan, then Senate majority leader Bill Frist, and conservative stalwarts such as Strom Thurmond and Orrin Hatch. Proponents of stem cell research depicted the White House as obstructing progress at every turn, delivering a lifetime of hardship, if not death, to millions of people who might otherwise be cured of inoperable conditions.

The Bush administration's use of children as a prop was neither accidental nor without precedent. They had been losing the public relations war, in part, because an opposing group of young people had been lobbying Congress for years to augment federal funding for stem cell research. Those children were members of the Juvenile Diabetes Research Foundation, now known simply as the JDRF, one of the most wide-reaching and influential advocacy groups in the healthcare industry.[1] The JDRF had been on the hunt for years, exhaustively lobbying the president and Washington's political elite about the urgency of investing in stem cell research. Years earlier the organization had invited President Bush and First Lady Laura Bush to be co-chairs of the Children's Congress, an event that brings young people to the Capitol to testify before the Senate about living with type 1 diabetes. The JDRF hoped that including the president would bridge the gap between his policy decisions and the grim realities confronting children with diabetes. The bald political maneuvering seemed warranted. After learning about the promise of stem cells at a closed-door Oval Office briefing, Bush stunned a senior health administrator when he reportedly commented, "Now I can see why these JDRF folks are so cranked up about this."[2] The organization was omnipresent, visiting members of Congress, being mentioned in White House press briefings, and gaining media visibility with their empathetic embodied activism. Unlike the American

Diabetes Association, which is a doctor-based organization, the JDRF is fueled by the experiences of children and parents who see bureaucratic road blocks as demonstrably fatal in a race for the cure. The JDRF is a fund-raising powerhouse, having raised approximately $1.7 billion for diabetes research as of this writing. The young activists fighting for their lives in forums such as the Children's Congress have garnered an impressive amount of media attention, as can be attested by the scores of news stories circulated about them annually.

In this chapter I investigate the rhetoric of the JDRF to contemplate how diabetes is culturally concocted as an essentially fatal disease. Unlike conceptions of management that imagine diabetes as easily controlled, the JDRF argues tirelessly that diabetes is sporadic, difficult to regulate, and eventually lethal. The group's organizers insist that diabetes is a source of bodily atrophy and suffering, not an ailment that can be readily governed. Arguing in opposition to voices that pose diabetes as surmountable, the JDRF contends that people with diabetes can be ever-mindful of their heath and still succumb to its ruinous consequences. Mindful that management discourses can be coopted by those not grappling with disease, the group posits emphatically that without federal assistance, diabetes is little more than a death sentence. This rhetoric is nowhere more pronounced than in the Children's Congress, a biannual gathering of hundreds of children with type 1 diabetes from around the country who gather on Capitol Hill and testify before Congress about the devastating effects of diabetes and the necessity to fund research that results in a cure. The fact that the JDRF can command a bipartisan congressional audience biannually speaks to its reach in Washington and the generative power of its rhetoric. Key to their appeal is a gracious ambivalence about the obligation to manage diabetes and advocate on their own behalf. For these kids, the reiterative rituals associated with diabetes are commensurate with a slow death that is a poor substitute for living free of chronic disease. Although many of them have access to technologies that keep their bodies in motion, the children predicate that they are on borrowed time in order to incite urgency about the need to cure diabetes.

The Children's Congress hearings are a mix of testimony from JDRF youth representatives and their parents, celebrities with personal or family connections to diabetes, scientists and health officials dedicated to curing the condition, and politicians who sit on the committee or have intimate investments in eradicating the disease. Prominently featuring the late Mary Tyler Moore, the celebrity face of type 1 diabetes for decades, the Children's Congress has garnered testimony from singers Tony Bennett and Nick Jonas, actors such as Kevin Kline and Jean Smart, astronaut James Lovell, and athletes such as Sugar Ray Leonard, Gary Hall, Jr., Adam Morrison, and Ray Allen. Some, such as Smart, Jonas, Morrison, and Hall, all live with diabetes. Others, such as Klein, Lovell, and Allen, have children with the condition. Each of them shares a tactical rhetoric that advocates for more resources, more care, and more awareness. They adopt an unyielding approach, insinuating that anything short of a cure perpetuates the daily suffering of children and a lifetime of unnecessary hardship.[3]

I examine testimony from the Children's Congress, beginning with its inception in 1999 through the year 2013. Most of the testimony (1999–2011) is taken directly from congressional databases. For as many years as possible I also watched video of the hearings, which were broadcast on C-SPAN or archived on the US Senate website.[4] The videos are indispensable, as they prevent reading the events as textual occasions devoid of the bodies of people demanding a cure. The hundreds of children gathered in the Capitol generally wear matching clothing and are seated on the floor space between the senators and the witness table where those participating in the event testify. This atmosphere has a profound effect on those involved, engendering affective bonds and emotive responses from the participants, including many US senators. Tears are shed often at the hearings, heartfelt promises are made by lawmakers, and real business is accomplished on Capitol Hill. The sessions facilitate an emotive repertoire of identification that inculcates research possibilities and fosters productive modes of stranger relationality between the children and their legislators. The very use of the phrase "the children" accomplishes much rhetorical work. As such, it is with "the children" that I shall begin.

Have You Checked the Children?

The "children" are a ubiquitous trope in the lexicon of America's political imaginary. Civic actors deploy the abstraction of "the children" similarly to the ways they might an empty signifier such as "the people," but with a hyperbolic emphasis on vulnerability, collective aspirations, and uncharted futures. Anita Bryant invoked "the children" as a metonym for a nation under assault by a villainous, if fabricated, predatory homosexual agenda. Forty years later, LGBT activist Dan Savage made a similar claim to "the children" to initiate a dialogue about shielding queer youth from the ominous and suffocating tentacles of heteronormativity. Though decidedly oppositional in their ideological orientation, nationalistic discourses punctuate each, projecting a utopic future that can be achieved only by rectifying the country's failure to realize communal ideals held by each of these political actors. The figure of the children, and its discursive accompaniment "the child," has been scrutinized widely in the humanities, and perhaps most explicitly in queer theory, to examine how youth are invoked to support policy platforms and mobilize draconian rhetorics of purity that seek to discipline and expunge LGBT people, racial minorities, and others from circumscribed characterizations of the nation.[5] Even when youth are articulated as non-normative, they are often situated in contradictory, though not necessarily counterintuitive, ways as disinterested assimilationists, radical separatists, and sometimes both simultaneously.[6] It is a time-honored American tradition to lament the supposed apathy of youth and the peril that awaits them, even as they are given little control over their own lives. Kathryn Boyd Stockton points out that children embody an unusual category of citizenship, occupying a precarious legal positionality that does not grant them full agency over the regulation of their desires or significant features of their everyday lives, such as their education.[7] Children exist largely outside the participatory mechanics of state politics and as such, their constitution in nationalistic rhetorics routinely reflects the political opportunism of their elders rather than any policies designed to better the future. Of course, the myriad ways children are made intelligible often speaks more to a culture's anxieties and hopes than it does any actual children.

In the fall of 1997, *Life* magazine ranked childhood as the fifty-fifth most important invention of the millennium, marking its advent in 1633 with the writings of Johan Amos Comenius. The magazine's emphasis on invention provides a stark reminder that how we envision childhood is not deterministically realized through age or dependency, but best conceived as a set of cultural constructs that have been shaped and reshaped for hundreds of years. In this way "childhood" might be thought of as the cumulative effect of social experimentation and shifting normativities, a rhetorical position that is guided as much by institutional negotiations as it is scripts of biological development or parenthood philosophies. The performative repertoires of childhood bestowed by society are not without their consequences. Critics such as Charles Morris remind us that the ways children are imagined in the public sphere limit the potency of their rhetorical performances.[8] Brian Amsden has likewise challenged critics to fully examine the ways in which teens and young adults complicate norms, lest we believe they are easily disciplined by bio-political normalization or are naïve products of liberal individualism.[9] In the words of danah boyd, the lives of children and teens are simply more complicated than our narratives allow them to be.[10] Still, everyone from psychologists to cultural critics appropriates the figure of the child to gauge hegemonic impulses and the dangers of cultural trends, such as new media technologies, rather than attending to the ways children exist in specific contexts. Children, especially as they morph into teenagers, are caricaturized in click-bait Facebook posts and on popular news sites as living examples of contradiction and puzzlement, being represented as both acting erratically and coming into consciousness to supersede obstacles. They are regarded as emotionally fungible, bemoaned by the generations ahead of them as being too apathetic, too stubborn, or too precocious. Their identities are imagined as necessitating room for individuality and the comforts of conformity. They want to fit in and be left alone. It is little wonder then that the experience of childhood is often positioned as a queer one.

The materiality of specific bodies, in this case those of young people with diabetes, necessarily alters the constitution and incorporation of "the children" in various nationalistic discourses. This has certainly been the case for children with diabetes, who have always occupied a pivotal space in the disease's genealogy. Prior to the discovery of insulin in 1922, children with type 1 diabetes generally died within a year of diagnosis— there was no hope of surviving to adulthood. After insulin was put to use, however, people were given a new lease on life, their bodies no longer wasting away from the biological inability to convert glucose to energy. Patients who were once emaciated and malnourished began regaining strength and appearing "normal," bringing hope to scores of families and medical practitioners. Photographs of children with diabetes both before and after insulin therapy were circulated widely to illustrate the resurrection effect enabled by the injectable substance. Indeed, generations of doctors were educated from textbooks that featured these pictures. As Chris Feudtner notes, the visual rhetoric of these photos had a dramatic effect on treatment and care, even if the promise that insulin would allow children with diabetes to live out the remainder of their "natural lives" without repercussions was overstated in initial reports.[11] The curative force of insulin suggested by the photos tended to overlook the technological revenge effects of hypoglycemia and the complications of living with a chronic disease. The photos also imparted a recurring theme in diabetes's history and one that is revisited in this chapter: that just under the surface of care lurks an incurable, predatory disease that necessitates vigilance, surveillance, and perpetual alarm. Such sentiments provide the rhetorical architecture for the JDRF's lobbying efforts and media campaigns when they descend on Capitol Hill.

The articulation of childhood with activism produces unique renderings of civic identity that rest outside typical frameworks of youth identity. If the varying delineations of childhood outlined at the start of this section constitute a normal trajectory of development, then child activists, especially those with disabilities, are atypical in their focused pursuits. It would be wrongheaded to allege that these children present yet another example of infantile citizenship, one that relegates the embodiment of disease to the figure of the child to spur action on the part of national actors. Contrary to that inclination, I believe JDRF delegates epitomize Lauren Berlant's now iconic notion of "diva citizenship." The youth representatives call into question the dominant narrative of the nation's commitment to childhood by repeatedly highlighting their exacerbating marginalization. They flip the script of normality and childhood—too easily coopted in Washington—to urge action, change, and the promise of a better tomorrow. The young advocates occupy a congressional space that is not designed for them—they cannot, after all, vote. Members of the Children's Congress confront those in power by asking why health care is not universal, why stem cell research is not fully funded, and why programs such as Medicare do not cover technologies that keep people alive. They feed the utopic impulse that "these acts of risky dramatic persuasion are based on a belief that the privileged persons of national culture will respond to the sublimity of reason."[12] This is not to say that every moment of the Children's Congress is a spectacular act that challenges the normative functions of governmentality.[13] Nonetheless, their work highlights how invocations of citizenship and disability can be strategically framed to address the failures of the US political system.

The Children's Congress presents an embodied disruption to the parlance of normative development generally tethered to national identity. Several of the minors featured in this chapter grapple with multiple ailments, not only diabetes but also conditions such as kidney failure. Their experiences of "growing sideways" trouble cultural ideals of individual responsibility, self-sufficiency, and personal sovereignty. They are compelled to educate adults about the limits of their bodies in the present and chart a future that may never materialize. In short, the coupling of chronic disease and youth personas produces subjectivities that rest outside the proscriptions of traditional management discourses. Unlike much work in queer studies that tends to segment discussions of disability from analyses of childhood, ambassadors to the JDRF elucidate a disruption of scripts that portend an auspicious future. Fatalism acts as a structuring mechanism for their rhetoric, disarming common assumptions about the capacity to manage disease and the fate that awaits them.

Of course, the Children's Congress might have the negative consequence of reiterating media representations of "super crips" or acting as "inspiration porn." They risk being situated as transcendent figures that provide comfort to those unaccustomed to their disabilities. Public narratives about the JDRF tend to replicate such portraits, principally focusing on a representative's ability to overcome obstacles and raise money. Even when the event features degrees of inspiration, however, fatalistic allusions quickly check any hope being imparted by the delegates. For every reparative move made by the children, there is always a lurking paranoia about the effects of disease, the perils of ignoring science, and the bleak future that awaits them without congressional action.

Courting Congressional Kin

When the Children's Congress first appeared on Capitol Hill in 1999, approximately 16 million Americans had some form of diabetes, with roughly 800,000 new cases being reported each year. At the time diabetes cost the country about $105 billion annually, and one out of every four Medicare dollars was spent treating the condition. By the time the JDRF lobbied Congress in 2013 the estimated number of Americans living with diabetes had soared to 29 million people, with more than eight million of those believed to be undiagnosed. Expenditures had climbed to $245 billion annually; one of every three Medicare dollars was now spent on diabetes-related complications. Despite ample warning that diabetes rates and costs were flooding the healthcare system, little was being done in Washington to patch the dam at the turn of the century. Congress reliably talked out of both sides of its mouth when addressing calls to fund medical research, even as it acknowledged a national crisis was imminent. Anticipating a deluge of diabetes diagnoses, for instance, the Senate passed a unanimous resolution to double appropriations for the National Institute of Health (NIH) in the mid-1990s. When the time came to actually allocate money for research, however, it voted down proposals in three consecutive sessions.[14] The JDRF became a critical player in resisting such duplicity, championing funding initiatives such as the Special Diabetes Program (SDP). The SDP provides millions of dollars in research funding but has required constant advocacy to remain solvent. In 2005, the congressionally mandated Diabetes Research Working Group reported that the SDP was funded at only 65 percent of its projected need, well short of the $1.6 billion recommended.[15] In an era when any federally sponsored program is left open to charges of big government run amok, the role of organizations such as the JDRF has become vital to securing and protecting resources that would lead to a cure.

The JDRF is especially adept at recognizing how the political winds are blowing in Washington and adjusting its sails to maintain a clear link between the organization's goals and shifting congressional priorities. The group adroitly tailors its advocacy efforts to specific political moments even as it is steadfast in maintaining its focus on finding a cure. Note the plasticity of their agenda: In 1999, Congress's failure to increase NIH funding compelled the JDRF to testify before the Senate Committee on Appropriations to register their dissent. In 2001, the JDRF found itself imploring the Bush administration to embrace stem cell research to further advancements that might lead to a cure. In 2003, the JDRF was dealing with the aftermath of the president's unpopular decision to withhold funds from such endeavors, and by 2007, stem cells had practically disappeared from their rhetoric as the organization aggressively pursued funding for the development of an artificial pancreas. In the wake of the Affordable Care Act's (ACA) implementation, participants testified before the Senate Committee on Aging, pushing for Medicare to fund continuous glucose monitors. More recently, they have attended to the hazards posed by the American Health Care Act. Of course, there is no magic bullet in politics, and no single organization is going to have a resolute impact on Congress. The cumulative result of political productivity comes from a mixture of opportunity, public opinion, organizational muscle, and cultural narratives that conform to the expectations of legislative possibility. Despite this recalcitrance, the clamoring of hundreds of children around the Capitol has a noticeable effect on policy makers.

Delegates to the JDRF are told repeatedly that their presence has a profound impact on deliberations about expenditure distribution because they "put a face" on an otherwise abstract issue. This sentiment was relayed by the now infamous foot-stomping senator Larry Craig of Montana, who beamed, "there are a good many choices and there are a lot of very necessary causes. But when all of you come and you are here and you visit with us, or your Senators, you put a face to the need. That helps us a great deal."[16] In 2005, Susan Collins told the JDRF, "all of us hear a lot of witnesses, hundreds and thousands of witnesses over the years that we have been Senators, but I don't think we have ever had a more compelling, persuasive group of witnesses than the panel we have just heard."[17] That same year Senator Frank Lautenberg, whose granddaughter has diabetes, joked with the participants about the empathy they impart: "I thank each one of you for the message that you bring us today. It causes us to look inside a little more deeply and to say, what is our responsibility here? Very seldom do we have hearings with witnesses, often business executives or scientists, and the tears that flow from those hearings are tears of boredom." The room erupted with laughter.[18] Lautenberg offered a particularly heartfelt message in 2005, just months after President Bush was sworn into office for a second term. He gushed:

> The fact is that we want to help, and I make a pledge to you here today that we will fight as hard as we can to see that there is more given to research

in this field and to stem cell research and to ask our colleagues . . . why can't we get a vote? If you could only hear these children, it would tell you enough to say, hey, listen, we find money to fight wars. We find money to defend ourselves against terror. There can be no greater terror in my mind than to find out that you have a child who has diabetes and what it entails in your life. So thank you. I love you all. Kisses.[19]

The drawbacks of framing health care as a combative mission that is brought to life using metaphors of war and terror is well rehearsed in both academic and public discussions of medicine.[20] Terms such as "battle" and "fight" often engender depression and guilt by implying that a person did not try hard enough to overcome disease or illness. And while such rhetoric has strong potential to interfere with patient agency when attending to disease, in the halls of Congress, especially with a Republican-controlled body, such language has at times produced opportunities for tapping into a discourse that generates identification with politicians who might otherwise remain unmoved. The year Lautenberg made the above plea the country was immersed in discussions about the use of torture to obtain information, the legal and moral implications of hastily invading a sovereign nation, and demystifying obtuse phrases such as "The War on Terror." In Lautenberg's analogy, lack of prevention is the terror and not necessarily the disease itself. Apathy—the lack of attention to the threat—is the real danger.

To be sure, the communions forged between members of the JDRF and their senators are not simply the product of enigmatic national imaginaries. Rather, they are initiated by connections among the participants, both young and old, who have firsthand experience with a life-altering ailment. A striking contextual component of these hearings includes testimony from public servants who profess to having relatives with diabetes, including many with type 1. Strom Thurmond had a daughter with type 1 diabetes and became an unlikely ally in the fight for embryonic stem cell research. Senators Jeanne Shaheen and Lautenberg both have grandchildren with type 1 diabetes and Senator Patty Murray has a niece with the condition. Other officials spoke about the effects diabetes had on their lives without being specific to type 1. Senator Carl Levin of Michigan told the committee in 2001 that he lost his best friend from law school to diabetes.[21] That same year, Senator Jean Carnahan commented that the hearings held particular meaning for her because her father suffered from the disease.[22] Senator Robert Bennett of Utah would echo this refrain about his grandfather two years later.[23] It is also not uncommon for senators to invoke firsthand experiences with diseases such as cancer during the gatherings.[24] The heartache cultivated by disease is ubiquitous among members of Congress, and they habitually articulate grief to the JDRF's aims. In a setting that is reliant on personal narrative, it is both decorous and oddly appropriate for senators to supply these intimate testimonials.[25]

The JDRF's success in bridging the gap between Republicans and Democrats is also noteworthy in a political culture that extols partisanship. Still, I would contend that it is not enough that these are child advocates. Politicians customarily vote against health care for the poor, increases in medical research, educational funding, gun control, and food stamp programs, all of which impact the lives of young people. As Collins noted in 2011, "In a government in which, too often, too little happens that is constructive these days, this is a cause that unites people across party lines and has enabled us . . . to come together to be supportive of diabetes research and to help facilitate some of the really miraculous advances that have occurred in dealing with diabetes in our time."[26] This optimistic take on the Children's Congress should not obscure the fact that these events are highly political and in many instances attached to issues particular to the needs of individual senators. Funding for the NIH, regulatory obstacles, and tax cuts have all been sources of contestation and consternation at the hearings.[27] In the face of this political labyrinth, the JDRF focuses relentlessly on the need for a cure and on the debilitating effects of diabetes. The Children's Congress constantly stresses the curative possibilities of research and the obstacles that prevent its members from living a normal life.

Cures, Complications, and the Rhetoric of Normality

The blasé style of Senate hearings all but guarantees that the slightest deviation from the norm can generate media attention. Hillary Clinton's retort to the Senate Foreign Relations Committee about an attack on a US embassy in Benghazi, Libya is a good example of how mild theatrics can garner immense public interest. We can find cognate examples in the words of Roger Gail Lyon, an AIDS activist who implored Congress to underwrite the resources necessary to combat the epidemic, saying, "This is not a political issue. This is a health issue. This is not a gay issue. This is a human issue. And I do not intend to be defeated by it. I came here today in the hope that my epitaph would not read that I died of red tape." Students of history will certainly recognize statements such as, "Have you no sense of decency, sir? At long last, have you left no sense of decency?" or "The central question at this point is simply put: what did the President know, and when did he know it?" The anticipatory, if sometimes humdrum, form of congressional testimony provides the means for participants to craft theatrics and political action in spectacular fashion. The JDRF is no exception, but with fewer moments of historical sublimity. Still, just as the most avid of congressional watchers can anticipate the ways probes will be directed at judicial nominees or politically scapegoated cabinet secretaries, the form of the Children's Congress is a genre replete with repetitive themes, tropes, and participants that provides a map for understanding the political action unfolding.

In this way, the Children's Congress is a study in form just as much as it is an analysis in content. Recurring motifs across the hearings reveal both strategic rhetorical choices and the deft ways these situations are navigated creatively by forum participants. The imitative features of the hearings, including the witnesses called to testify, the government emissaries present, and the media narratives that mark these children as exceptional, demarcate expectations among participants, permit a sense of accomplishment, and craft a continuity that fosters relationships from event to event. Variation exists among remarks, but there is enough rhetorical consistency that patterns of speech become decidedly noticeable. In many years, for example, the hearings have included a reference to the number of children diagnosed daily with type 1 diabetes (about thirty-five). For four consecutive appearances it was mentioned at the start of the hearing that diabetes is a leading contributor to kidney failure, blindness, amputation, and heart disease. The Children's Congress is made up of youngsters from across the nation, but those testifying almost always hail from the home states of sitting committee members. Because Senator Collins has taken the lead in the fight for type 1 diabetes research, a constituent from Maine has testified six of the eight times the JDRF took to Capitol Hill during the scope of this study.[28] The serial nature of the events outlines presuppositions among those contributing to the conversation and establishes a fluid alliance between the organization and politicians, especially for those managing concurrent business items in the Senate during the hearings.

Ambassadors to the Children's Congress emphasize the themes of hardship and discipline, continually accentuating the urgency associated with finding a cure. Politicians, scientists, parents, and children all repeat the rallying cry that "insulin is not a cure" to displace the prominence of management paradigms that might eclipse their message of ending the disease. Unlike optimistic public avowals about management, those participating in the hearings actively marginalize blithe sensibilities about diabetes. The motif that "medicine is not a cure" is ubiquitous, shaping every aspect of the JDRF's rhetorical corpus. In 1999, Mary Tyler Moore previewed this theme, arguing that medical interventions are crucial, but technologies are nothing more than a stopgap. "You know insulin is not a cure, as will the 30,000 children who will be diagnosed this year with diabetes. What gives us all hope at JDF is the promise of research and the commitment of this committee . . . to make doubling the NIH budget over the next five years a top priority."[29] For five consecutive sessions over the next decade, Collins announced to the committee in her opening remarks that insulin is not a cure.[30] These words were reiterated in 2001 by Senator Daniel Akaka, Jim Lovell, and Allen Spiegel, the former director of the National Institute of Diabetes and Digestive and Kidney Diseases at the NIH.[31] The phrase stretched to 2007 when it was again recited by Adam Morrison, delegate Caroline McEnery, and parent Ann Strader;[32] in 2009 by Nick Jonas and parent Ellen Gould;[33] and in 2011 by delegate Kerry Morgan.[34]

Giving presence to the shortcomings of medicine deflects contrarian predispositions about the ease of diabetes management and the capability of the children to traverse side effects. In doing so, the hearings provide a platform for crafting a sense of alarm in a notoriously slow legislative body. Mary Tyler Moore displayed prowess in this regard, ardently proving to be a remarkable advocate for the JDRF. Note the consistent use of imperative language in her testimony about life with diabetes:

> It means I have been *forced* to test my blood sugar several times a day and give myself multiple injections of insulin just to stay alive, day after

day after day. It means I have been *ripped awake* more times than I care to recall in a state of *extreme distress* caused by *life-threatening* low blood sugars. Ask my husband, Robert, who wakes up with me in the middle of the night to help me *fight* our 24-hour-a-day *battle* . . . The difficulties that I have experienced are reflected in each of these children who have had their childhood *stolen* from them and who have been *forced* to contemplate a *difficult* and *uncertain* future that may all too soon include similar *complications*.[35]

Unlike management frames that provide explanatory power—if not comfort—to those living free of diabetes, the condition here seems to be declaring open season on the children. The suffering imparted by Moore speaks to the resources children with type 1 diabetes require to stave off an arduous death. Her words prevent an easily adopted notion of diabetes as a condition that is effortlessly controlled, instead personifying it as combative and demanding vigorous surveillance to tame it. Again, such language might be counterproductive in a medical setting where militaristic lexicons sometimes prove to do more harm than good, but it is effective among political actors motivated by exigent threats. Likewise, in 2009 parent Ellen Gould, who has four children with type 1 diabetes, contrasted the necessity of a cure with the struggles confronting her family:

> While insulin therapy helps us manage this disease, insulin is not a cure. On many occasions, we carefully measure blood sugars, count carbohydrates, and inject what we think is just the right amount of insulin. And it is so discouraging when we measure just a few hours later and their blood sugar is way above the normal range. How many high blood sugars are too many? When will the long-term complications with their eyes, kidneys, or heart start to show? Sometimes we have to deal with the low blood sugars, like the Saturday morning several months ago when we were awakened by Sam, who had collapsed in his room, incoherent, because of a dangerously low blood sugar. It took us 20 minutes to get him back to normal. What happens the next time if we do not hear him?[36]

The fatalism implied in the testimony is neither hyperbolic nor trite. It reinforces that action must be taken in order for these children's lives to be saved.

The looming dangers of diabetes are actualized through disquieting metaphors that challenge understandings of diabetes as unhurried in its manifestation. Among the fiercest of these figures is that of the "time bomb," which has been used recurrently over the years. In 2001, for example, Moore signified diabetes as a "personal time bomb which can go off today, tomorrow, next year, or ten years from now, a time bomb affecting millions, like me and the children here today."[37] The metaphor was brought to life during a segment of Moore's testimony about a thirty-one-year-old woman named Danielle Alberti, who died on a flight to Australia.[38] The imagery of a bomb, on a plane, in the months before 9/11 may feel disconcerting in retrospect. Nonetheless, the rhetoric functions to retort preconceived ideas about diabetes's creeping ramifications. Gradualism can mean many things, but the erratic and explosive nature of a bomb replaces the slothfulness of everyday life with imagery that demands immediate action.[39]

The axiom that medicine is not a cure, the explosive metaphors employed by the JDRF, and the dislodging of management as a replacement for a cure all reinforce a stated desire for these children to live a "normal" life. This rhetoric stresses an assimilative longing among the participants by centralizing illness as a barrier to normalcy. The JDRF embraces the notion of normality as a strategic goal, consistently highlighting the failure of the body to function properly and, as a result, act as an impediment to socialization. Unlike some disabled cultures that embrace non-normative identifications, including many deaf communities who rebuff technologies such as cochlear implants, the JDRF unremittingly reiterates the ways science and technology are useful only to the extent that they allow people to arrive at a place of normality. At the first hearing Moore implored the committee to think through the terrible side effects that accompany life with diabetes. She argued, "To add to the day in and day out hassles of living with diabetes, the balancing of diet and exercise and insulin, the shots, the terrible episodes of low sugar, the debilitating feelings of high sugars is the knowledge that even if you do all you can to be normal, you're not. You're different and you face the uncertainty of an adulthood visited upon by early blindness, kidney failure, amputation, heart attack or stroke."[40] The bodily limitations brought about by diabetes prevent the children from reaching benchmarks that constitute ordinary life both in the present and the foreseen future. Enthymematically, the only possibility that hoists them into the orbit of a normal life is a cure.

Representatives to the Children's Congress rarely narrate diabetes as easily managed, choosing instead to detail a life rife with struggle, suffering, difference, and danger. Speaking of the delegates in 2003, Moore cautioned the senators, "don't be misled by their drive, their energy, and their unwavering commitment. They—and I—struggle every minute of every day to do what happens naturally for people who don't have diabetes."[41] She continues, "Each of these children and I need to be a mathematician, a physician, a personal trainer, and a dietitian all rolled into one."[42] Pointing to the statistics about complications she contended, "I have seen studies that say that virtually everyone with juvenile diabetes shows evidence of heart disease by age 40—and, further, that the premenopausal women with juvenile diabetes have a more than 30 times greater risk of death from heart attack."[43] If management were an effective tool on its own merits, there would be fewer deaths and only mild repercussions—but such is not the case and the organization pursues that thesis aggressively. Anything short of a cure is unconscionable.

Appeals that use the trope of normality are especially potent coming from children who communicate the desire to simultaneously blend in with their peers but also perform cultural scripts of individuality. Normality is an especially persuasive device in front of a congressional audience that not only feels accountable to its young constituents, but who are guided time and again by conventional rhetorics that range from public opinion polls to political vernacular extolling "common sense." The notion of normality surfaces time and again, as when sixteen-year-old delegate Asa Kelly testifies, "A cure would give us freedom to carry on a *normal* life without taking a break to check our blood or have a snack. I want Congress to feel the urgency of this issue—that it is a daily struggle, not just something we can take a break from doing. It is our life style and all choices are made due to it."[44] Aaron Jones, age ten, noted that he sometimes has seizures as a result of his diabetes. "Living with diabetes is the pits. I live with it because I have to. The part I really don't like is taking insulin shots and always checking my blood sugar. It can be painful sometimes. I just don't feel like doing it. I also feel awful and tired when my blood sugars get too high or very low. I just want to feel like a *normal* kid without pricking my fingers 2,000 times each year or injecting myself with insulin 1,100 times a year."[45] Pleas for normality are not always stated directly but communicated through mundane experiences such as attending a birthday party or participating in team sports. Seventeen-year-old Caroline McEnery told the committee, "I knew that with each meal came a needle, with each birthday party, a sugar-free cake, and with each good night to my parents, the worry about a low blood sugar episode during the night. More than anything, I knew that I would be different than all of my friends."[46] Children's Congress representative Will Smith from New York City testified that he loved sports and dreams of a professional career. But he also told the committee that it is "painful not to have the freedom of eating whatever I want. While other kids can eat pizza or cheeseburgers whenever they're hungry, I have to consider how those might push up my blood sugar readings too high."[47] Far from the mundane experiences of childhood, some participants give heartbreaking accounts of having to grow up too fast. Tré Hawkins, a twelve-year-old from Detroit, told the committee that diabetes "has been a financial burden on my grandparents and my mom, but they try hard to make my life as normal as possible and they don't complain."[48] At every turn normality escapes these kids, be it through the sociality of eating, the relationality of teen rituals, or the discrepancies of economic structures. Many of them are "growing sideways," to borrow a phrase from Stockton, saddled with adult responsibilities and occupying a temporality that is divergent from their peers.

The struggle to achieve normality is regularly partnered with a discourse that exalts the promise of a cure and the radical impact such a discovery would have on the lives of the participants. In 2003, Sophia Cygnarowicz told the committee, "I don't know what life is like without diabetes, but I sure would like to find out. Finding a cure is important to me because I won't have to take shots or do blood tests. Most of all, I could eat a Sno-Cone whenever I wanted to. My friends in this room and I aren't asking for much. We just want a life without diabetes."[49] A number of students divulged that their blood sugars are capricious and not easily reined in by management regimens. Nine-year-old Stockton Morris disclosed the cumbersome side effects diabetes has on his body: "I get dizzy, go limp and can't get up. They tell me this will have a bad effect on my body down the road. Low blood sugar is not good for my brain. It will be awesome for a cure. I'd love not having to do blood sugar tests."[50] Mollie Singer, a ten-year-old delegate from Nevada, didn't even trust hospital staff, who seemed to lack the experience to treat her sugars. She testified, "A year after I got diabetes I had open heart surgery and I had a real bad time. When I was in the hospital no one knew how to handle a child with diabetes and I got the wrong amount of insulin and the wrong food."[51] At every turn another time bomb needs to be defused.

The desire among the participants to assimilate sometimes came at the expense of closely monitoring their health and maintaining rituals that would preclude aftereffects. Management requires a highly cognizant and vigilant patient to ensure that disease does not overrun the body. Children and teenagers, already considered rebellious and noncompliant, become familiar figures of transgression when medicine is factored into the equation. Several of the delegates testified to discarding their routines, finding such practices too restrictive for their hectic lives. Fifteen-year-old Rachel Dudley remembered:

> Several times a day, my mom would ask if I had checked my blood sugar level and if I had taken my insulin. I would always tell her what she wanted to hear, even though I sometimes ignored my blood sugar reading and injected the wrong amount of insulin. Occasionally, I even injected the insulin into the toilet, instead of into my arm. Looking back, I simply did not want to have diabetes, and I thought that I could be like a normal kid by simply ignoring the necessity of my daily routine.[52]

Individual maintenance is critical to staving off diabetes's consequences, and young people who struggle with the disease exacerbate the need for a cure. The cumbersome emotional weight of living with diabetes can generate feelings of denial and helplessness, eventually leading to guilt and shame. Teens are not alone in these self-sabotaging activities, but their public declarations about nonconformity amplify the exigent circumstances that demand a cure.

The futility of management and the quest to find a cure were further reinforced by representatives whose health was already being lethally compromised. Laniece Evans Scott, who was ten at the time of her testimony and had been diagnosed at sixteen months, had experienced especially extreme complications. "I was diagnosed with juvenile diabetes after going into a coma when I was only sixteen months old. I spent the first five years of my life in and out of hospitals. My mom had to learn how to give me shots and take care of me. She has not been able to work because she has to take care of me all the time. She drives me five hours to see a special doctor who helps me care for my diabetes."[53] Eleven-year-old Caroline Rowley of Houston, quoted in the epigraph of this chapter, recounted a sobering story about a blind woman coming into her school to discuss seeing-eye dogs. Because the woman had mentioned giving herself shots, Caroline surmised that the visitor had diabetes. "When I got home, I asked my Mom if we would get a new dog or train our dog, Chase, to be my eyes when I went blind."[54] She remembered, "My Mom sat me down, and with tears in her eyes, she told me we were going to do everything in our power to keep me from getting complications." Years later Caroline discovered she was in the beginning stages of kidney disease. She implored the committee: "When is this all going to stop? I always thought that if I ever got complications, that I would be grown, but I would still have my youth to be normal, but diabetes has stolen my childhood and forced me to grow up. I worry about having a seizure, going blind or losing my kidneys. The top-ten music countdown or the latest fashions at Gap, these things just do not seem that important in my life."[55] Many of these kids have suffered injuries enough for multiple lifetimes. The present they occupy is dreary and the future affords little hope. When Senator Collins asked eighteen-year-old Eric Bonness what the hardest part of having diabetes is, he replied, "I would have to say that no matter how careful you think you are, how much care you are taking with your diabetes, your sugars are always off. There is always something that—you can never have total control, which means you are going to end up having complications. So just the fear of not being able to fully be in control of this disease is probably the most scary thing."[56] The dialectic between superfluous management and the terrifying abyss of uncontrollable diabetes is communicated incessantly across the hearings. Some of the young ambassadors testified that they test their blood sugar up to eighteen times a day.[57] Others recall losing their glucose monitor 300 miles away from home, leaving them to guess their blood sugar levels prior to taking insulin—a precarious position to occupy in unfamiliar settings.[58] Diabetes is burdensome both when one is at the top of one's game and when circumstances are out of one's control. And, for all of the strides made in diabetes care, management is not a cure.

Diabetes is especially perilous when the children are confronted by others who are ignorant of the disease and its menacing ramifications. This included not only the children's peers, but also adults who mistakenly stress the import of individual fortitude over medical realities. Andrew Webber of Steep Falls, Maine told the committee he was embarrassed to test his blood sugars and take shots in front of his baseball team. "Last year in Little League, I was having many abnormal blood sugars. My coaches did not understand how diabetes works, so they assumed that I was goofing off and I needed to take breaks. Instead of listening to my parents and allowing me the time to recover, they chose to bench me. I got a reputation for being uncooperative."[59] Close contacts often graph the most challenging elements of disease management onto the personalities of the kids themselves, inadvertently projecting a lack of control as a moral failure. A cure is needed to save them not simply from the destructiveness of diabetes, but from the social stigma imposed by other people. One teen, Katie Halasz, frightfully disclosed that school administrators will allow her blood to be tested only in the nurse's office, requiring her to descend two flights of stairs while experiencing hypoglycemia. She lamented:

> Some of my teachers think that I leave the classroom just to get out of class. Do they think I enjoy sticking a needle in my finger? When my blood sugars are high, I cannot concentrate on my work and my vision gets blurred. My teachers do not understand. Some of them even think it is my fault that my sugars go high because they think that I eat things like candy bars. They do not understand that my sugars can go up for no apparent reason. Educating my teachers has been my biggest challenge since being diagnosed with diabetes.[60]

Likewise, Scott heartbreakingly told the committee, "I have a lot of trouble in school because the teachers send me home when my blood sugar levels are bad. I am not bad. I am good. It is the diabetes that is bad. I do the best I can, but I am only a kid and diabetes is a horrible disease. I have fallen behind in school because I miss so many classes."[61] Persistently dealing with uneducated adults contributes to a hazardous environment that lends an air of instability wherever the kids may be. These accounts are spectacular on their own merits and are powerful sources of evidence when reviewed as a collection.

The JDRF amasses these representative anecdotes and conjoins them with familiar medical regimens to present them as a quasi-form of aggregate data. Michel Foucault postulated that the use of assessment tools, such as statistical data, at the end of the nineteenth century helped to formulate a normal subject whose desires and needs can be carefully plotted.[62] This crafting of normality is especially powerful in health and medicine, as everything from the BMI to the Kinsey scale is conceived around numerical data. A typical rhetorical strategy for the Children's Congress is to convey degrees of (non)normality through the recitation of statistics about the regularity of shots and finger pricks that the kids perform on a continual basis. Although it is common today to discuss individual identity being lost to amalgamations of data, the JDRF utilizes statistics to give presence to the confounding medical problems that plague individual children. In 1999 Singer revealed to the committee, "I am ten years old and I have had diabetes since 1993. In the past 5½ years I have taken 8,395 shots of insulin and I have poked my fingers 20,987 times. Everything I do is planned around my diabetes—eating, sleeping, playing, and even homework. If things are not planned exactly, my blood sugar levels can go out of control."[63] Cygnarowicz had just finished first grade when she appeared before Congress. She had been grappling with diabetes since she was just a year old and testified, "I have taken 4,380 shots of insulin and have pricked my finger over 13,000 times to test my blood sugar. I don't like it. It hurts. It is so hard to keep my blood sugar in a good range. No matter how hard I try, I still go low and high."[64] One of the most effective uses of this strategy was employed by thirteen-year-old Lauren Stanford, who expounded:

> I want you to think about something. In this room right now, you see 150 kids with juvenile diabetes. That is 150 pairs of hands. Consider that, on average, each of these kids needs to prick their finger and draw blood for a glucose test six times a day. Add to that the fact that we have each had juvenile diabetes for an average of five years. If you do the math, you will see that this means that there are 150 pairs of hands that prick their fingers more than 1.5 million times and have spent over $2 million on just

their test strips. If you look out into this hearing room, you will see the evidence of the 1.5 million times that diabetes has invaded a life. And we are just a snapshot of the millions of kids who suffer with diabetes. So take my story that I am about to share with you and multiply it just like we did those finger pricks and you will begin to understand the toll this disease takes on our world.[65]

The JDRF uses tools that could be culled directly from a public speaking textbook: They ordinarily use statistics and examples in their testimony to enrich their credibility with the right balance of empathy and rationality. The emphasis on normality, the reiteration of painful rituals, the broadcasting of statistics, and the ignorance of those surrounding the children all convey an exigence that can be met only through a cure. And for that they turn to scientists who confirm the grim future that awaits them should Congress remain unmoved.

Scientific Ethos and the Prospects of Embodied Activism

The disquieting alarm pervasive in the JDRF's appeals is effective only to the extent that it offers lawmakers opportunities to fund a cure and curtail the hardship children with diabetes experience. The most expedient course of action is to direct resources into scientific endeavors that might revitalize the pancreas or technologies that act as a stopgap until a cure is developed. The search for a cure, be it the experimentation that led to the discovery of insulin or the slow progress that has been made on an artificial pancreas, has necessarily depended on major investments in science and medicine that produce refined treatments. And there is no sponsor of scientific research more prominent than the federal government. Just as the JDRF has exhibited prowess in monitoring political shifts in Washington, it has been equally proficient in surveying and sponsoring scientific activity that might result in a cure. To ground the appeals made by members of the Children's Congress, the JDRF incorporates testimony from scientists who bestow plausibility to narratives accentuating the end of diabetes. Although fatalism is an essential component of the JDRF's rhetoric, attention to science endows solvency to an otherwise decrepit reality. The contemporary telos of diabetes is death, but scientific intervention professes a new hope, one that reinforces nationalistic impulses to protect children, combat disease, and elevate the prominence of science. As a result, hearings generally feature medical undertakings and the promise such research holds for eliminating type 1 diabetes. Over the years, conversations at the hearings have included topics such as genetics and genomics, cell communication, neuropathies, stem cells, GAD protein cells, and immune tolerance, among others. This section focuses on two of the most significant undertakings made by the JDRF—the fight to bolster stem cell research and the pursuit of the artificial pancreas.

Championing these advocacy efforts served multiple functions, not only fostering the possibility of extending the lives of people with diabetes, but also inviting politicians in the chamber to join the cause by leaning on lethargic government agencies and acting as witnesses to technological innovations. Although discussions concerning stem cells were couched in spectacular rhetorics about the resurrection of internal organs, and the artificial pancreas portends a cyborg body not yet realized, each reinforces the desperate need for a cure and the prospect of a life better lived. Appeals for augmented stem cell research proved to be politically precarious, whereas the technological promise of the artificial pancreas was met with universal approval. Discussions about each of these treatments also suggested that the United States was falling behind other countries such as Canada, where progress on both items accelerated rapidly. The gradualism of the disease and the bureaucratic process were slowly encroaching on the children.

The Lazarus Effect: Stem Cells and Life After a Slow Death

Few technologies in modern endocrinology have been met with greater public enthusiasm than stem cell research. Although tools such as insulin pumps have become familiar instruments for managing diabetes, they stop short of being curative and have received mixed reviews from both patients and doctors.[66] Stem cells, however, have the potential to radicalize treatment, becoming a medical marvel for tens of thousands of patients globally. The excitement generated by stem cell transplants was considerable among JDRF advocates, who expended immense cultural capital rallying congressional leaders about the science's inspired potential. Health officials such as Dr. Harold Varmus, then head of the

NIH, argued at the 1999 Children's Congress that stem cells were one of the most auspicious advancements in the fight against type 1 diabetes.[67] The Bush administration's refusal to engage the uncharted opportunities of stem cells led the JDRF to embrace the issue, knowing full well they had the support of the American public and their respective legislators. Nonetheless, the move by the White House to frame stem cells in moral and not scientific terms obstructed scientific innovations and with it the hopes of millions of people living with chronic conditions. As John Lynch has persuasively observed, by eschewing scientific idioms, "Bush set aside a mode of public deliberation that allows for linking real definitions with ideological commitments" and inhibited attempts at crafting a coherent political compromise.[68] The JDRF was able to elicit sympathy from Congress, but the president remained unmoved by their struggles.

In retrospect, the progress made on stem cells by the JDRF, in conjunction with cognate advocacy groups, seems as gradual as the disease they were fighting to cure. For every victory there were setbacks and for every vote they cultivated there loomed the threat of a presidential veto. Despite these drawbacks, the campaign marked a significant milestone for the group, which helped to bring about votes in both chambers of Congress. Collins called stem cell research "the issue of the day" at the 2001 Children's Congress, the same year the JDRF pressed for legislation that would fund stem cell research for the next four years.[69] The JDRF did have some success corralling support for human islet transplants, which proved to be less controversial than stem cell therapies. Although islet transplants are *not* the same as stem cell transplants, the issues were often discussed in close proximity because of the regenerative potential of each.[70] Thanks to the JDRF's efforts, fifty-two senators signed the Pancreatic Islet Cell Transplantation Act, which was passed unanimously by both the House and Senate and signed into law by President Bush.[71] The bill, however, was limited in reach, dealing mainly with the donation of cadaver pancreases and mild oversight regulations. The measure also constrained the ability of scientists to perform useful research. As Dr. Hugh Auchincloss, Professor of Surgery at Massachusetts General Hospital and Harvard Medical School, told the Senate, "Even if we used every available cadaver donor pancreas for islet transplantation, we would have only enough islets to cure 0.1 percent of all people with type 1 diabetes. That is the number that I want people to remember, 0.1 percent of people with type 1 diabetes."[72] The underwhelming impact of the legislation caused the JDRF to rally, returning to the issue for the next two hearings, even if the promise of stem cell technology remained obscured by Bush's political malfeasance. Notwithstanding the roadblocks established by the president, the scientific community held on to the hope that a cure might be around the corner. Spurred in part by the news that a dozen people in Canada had been cured of type 1 diabetes through islet cell transplants, advocates lobbied vigorously to import this breakthrough to the United States.[73]

The miraculous narratives that accompanied islet transplants provided compelling testimony about the potential of science to regenerate the production of insulin in the body and render diabetes obsolete. Dr. Allen Spiegel presented evidence of success from the Transplantation and Autoimmunity Branch of the National Institute of Diabetes and Digestive and Kidney Diseases of the NIH Clinical Center. In 2001 he told the story of a fifty-seven-year-old woman who had been living with type 1 diabetes for more than fifty years and who was cured, at least temporarily, using islet transplants.[74] He described her as a "brittle diabetic" whose sugars were "wildly abnormal." After the transplants, however, her sugars had stabilized, leading her to become insulin-free.[75] Even though this was still relatively anecdotal from a scientific perspective, eradicating diabetes in a person who lived with it for five decades was nothing to sneer at. The promise of a cure was far more persuasive than the debilitating realities of management. If the disease need not be fatal, the logic went, surely political actors would be motivated to act. Such did not prove to be the case.

Although statistical data were years off, the reports of patients who had received islet transplants and who were living independent of insulin were astounding. In 2003, Dr. Bernhard Hering, director of Islet Transplantation at the University of Minnesota, testified about Lorna, a thirty-five-year-old mother of two who developed diabetes at age nine. Lorna lost her ability to sense that her blood sugar was dropping and her severe hypoglycemia led to a number of life-altering consequences. Lorna was stripped of her driver's license, fired from her job, divorced, and had visitation privileges with her children revoked. Scientific innovation transformed her life. Lorna entered the hospital for a short procedure and an infusion that took roughly twenty minutes. She was kept for observation for two days and then released. The audience listened intently as Hering described "the Lazarus effect" on her life:

> Lorna's blood sugar levels returned to normal. She was able to completely discontinue insulin injections one month after her islet transplant. Since her transplant, she has not experienced a single episode of severe hypoglycemia. She learned to love life again, rediscovered her ability to make contributions to our world, regained control over her destiny, received her driver's license back, found a new job, married the paramedic who had repeatedly saved her life while she was diabetic.[76]

The audience erupted. Hering continued over the excitement, "She closed on a new home, and was granted authorization to take care of her boys again, all in the first year after her transplant. Now, almost three years later, Lorna continues to be insulin independent and diabetes free."[77] The testimony appeared persuasive to everyone involved, save the Bush administration.

The JDRF capitalized on this movement, imploring Congress to pass the Castle-Doggett Stem Cell Research Enhancement Act, the bill mentioned at the start of the chapter that was eventually vetoed by the president.[78] The administration's obstruction animated the JDRF's rhetoric and the group pointed time and again to the calamitous effects that would result from the executive decision. The JDRF revisited the chilling effects of this judgment for years. In 2005, Moore returned to the trope of fatalism in her testimony, beseeching the committee to take action and dramatizing diabetes's dire consequences should nothing be done: "As the Senate debates and votes on this stem cell bill, I ask you to remember us. Remember the stories we tell about injections, blood tests, about seizures, blindness, kidney failure, heart attack, amputations and strokes, about tearful nights and worrying parents, about lives altered wholly and completely, about what a cure really means to me and these courageous delegates and the millions just like us."[79] Management, for all of its benefits, is accompanied by pain and agony and is most assuredly no substitute for a cure. But the White House's unilateral decision to block funding for stem cell research above the objections of Congress presented insurmountable hurdles.[80]

Four years later, Douglas Wick, a film producer and co-head of Red Wagon Entertainment, recounted his daughter Tessa's journey with diabetes. In his recollections, the disease tarnishes every element of family life, from evening dinners to banal memories. Wick's testimony was perhaps most compelling because he discussed his close relationship with Nancy Reagan and their shared support of stem cell research. Reagan's backing was always particularly powerful because she watched Alzheimer's wreak havoc on her husband's health. Wick painfully recalls when the president decided to stunt progress and further endanger his daughter's life. "The day President Bush was to announce his position on federal funding for stem cell research, our whole family sat around the TV waiting. As the President announced his new policy, my wife, who always kept her chin up for the children, started to cry."[81] The scene presented is rife with traditional values: a family gathered around the television for an important government announcement, a reliant maternal figure breaking down, and the looming presence of Ronald Reagan. In this scenario, however, Wick and the former first lady are but ordinary citizens standing helpless before an administration who put ideological purity above the scientific frontier. Emotions were high because one avenue for a cure, perhaps the best one in diabetes's long history, had been foreclosed.

Focusing on stem cells was vexed by the ceaseless necessity to dispel myths about its scientific parameters. This included the frequent conflation with cloning, which was a non sequitur deployed by the White House to generate public sympathy for its stance. It never worked. Public support for stem cell research remained high. Scientists were also required to explain that embryos from in vitro fertilization are generally discarded if not used.[82] Further, much of the early research being investigated with pluripotent stem cells cultivated from embryos was being conducted in the private sector, leaving government officials in the dark when it came to medical advancements.[83] Recognizing their pleas were not having the desired effect, the JDRF refocused its efforts on funding for the artificial pancreas.

The Artificial Pancreas and the Approximation of a Cure

The phrase "artificial pancreas" evinces images from science fiction of cyborg entities whose chimeric character represents the future of the human race. The realities of an artificial pancreas are decidedly less fantastic, even if they do portend a promising future for people with diabetes. At this time, there is no device that holds the distinction of being such an apparatus—that is, a machine that can accurately read blood sugars along with the dispensation of insulin *and* glucose as needed by the body. The closest technology we have to the artificial pancreas is a closed-loop system that employs an insulin pump and a continuous glucose monitor (CGM) that work together to chart a person's sugar levels. The CGM takes multiple glucose readings every minute and then communicates electronically with the pump to regulate sugars. Unlike shots, which require a degree of prudence to master, CGMs process sugars automatically and are especially useful for avoiding severe nighttime lows that plague many people with diabetes. If sugars drop dramatically, CGMs can detect descending levels and the pump will curtail the amount of insulin being administered. Although science is getting closer to perfecting the dispensation of insulin, the burden of separately delivering glucose, not to mention the proper balancing of the two substances, has proven more difficult. Because the machines approximate the operations of the pancreas, the closed-loop system is as close to a proxy for a cure as we have, even if an imperfect one. Early studies have suggested that people with type 1 diabetes using closed-loop systems are at lower risk for heart disease, kidney failure, and sight degeneration.[84]

Testimony focusing on the artificial pancreas was relatively mundane, especially when contrasted with the miraculous nature of stem cells. Despite the lackluster rhetoric used to describe the device, it created an occasion for the JDRF to flex its political muscle. This was on display most explicitly at the 2011 hearing, which exposed a noticeable frustration with the Food and Drug Administration (FDA). The notoriously slow agency was accused of moving at a glacial pace in approving technologies connected to the artificial pancreas. In what proved to be the most awkward exchange in the history of the Children's Congress, members of the Senate sparred with Chip Zimliki, chairman of the Artificial Pancreas Critical Path Initiative, located within the Center for Devices and Radiological Health at the FDA. Zimliki, himself a person with type 1 diabetes, had the difficult task of representing this oft unpopular branch of government while surrounded by hundreds of children.[85] Zimliki insisted that the FDA was doing its best within the parameters of the law to get new technologies to the market and was not being intentionally obstructionist.[86] He assured the crowd, "As a person with diabetes, I am acutely aware of the benefits an artificial pancreas system will provide. I say 'will' because I am highly optimistic that industry, researchers, and the FDA will bring this device to market."[87] Zimliki dutifully communicated the FDA's efforts, including an accelerated program that allowed a software developer working on the artificial pancreas to maneuver around a year's worth of regulatory obstacles.[88] Expedited as that process may have been, the ambiguity inherent in some of Zimliki's claims left the audience wanting more. The proxy cure provided by the artificial pancreas appeared to be tangled in red tape.

Senators participating in the event were not moved by Zimliki's personal appeals or institutional assurances. Collins pointed to a letter signed by fifty-nine members of the Senate offering guidance to the FDA for moving forward on the approval of the artificial pancreas. She also could not fathom why cognate technologies were available in Canada, but not stateside. Just as legislatures had raised the issue of Canada experimenting with stem cell therapies a decade earlier, it was again brought to the committee's attention that their neighbors to the north seemed to be making more efficient and promising scientific strides than they were.[89] Zimliki worked to clarify the differences between the two countries' regulatory systems, but the 200 children flanking him mitigated administrative explanations. Senator Mark Begich of Alaska pressed Zimliki, wanting to know why government regulations were standing in the way of advancements: "You said you were working through that, and no disrespect, but when I have Federal folks in front of me, it is always, 'soon,' 'maybe,' 'we are working on it.'"[90] Senator Scott Brown observed that there were 255 medical device companies in his then home state of Massachusetts, including the powerhouse Medtronic, and they continually pointed to the FDA as an inefficient body that hampered medical progress.[91] Like Collins, Brown also noted that these devices were approved in countries such as Ireland and he was perplexed as to why they were not being manufactured in the States. The audience met Brown's statement with applause.[92]

By the time Senator Shaheen, whose granddaughter has diabetes, was given the floor, Zimliki was clearly unsettled. Shaheen shared her colleagues' frustrations, but also assured Zimliki she was pleased to learn that the FDA would be charting a path for development. However, when she inquired into the next steps for approving the device, Zimliki retorted, "Can you clarify which artificial pancreas type system you are asking about?"[93] In other settings his question would merit dialogue, but in this space, on this occasion, it felt ill timed. When the FDA spokesperson began discussing the Veo insulin pump, which is not an artificial pancreas, Shaheen fired back:

> I appreciate that. I think for many of the people in this audience, they do not see that as the artificial pancreas that we are really hoping will be on the market. I agree, that is a step in the right direction, but as has been pointed out, that device is available on the market in other countries, and we would like to see not only that device available here, but to go to the next step, to have a continuous system available for people.[94]

I underline this exchange not to accuse one agency, and certainly not one individual with diabetes, with single-handedly inhibiting progress on care. Rather, I want to underscore the reach of the JDRF and the support its rhetoric engenders. The organization pushes hard on a powerful government agency with the help of sitting senators, even if those legislators have conflicting rationales for rebuking the FDA or see political gain for doing so. Brown was concerned about businesses in his state, while Mark Pryor focused on the costs of technologies for middle-class families, and Begich on bureaucratic obstructionism. Although it is easy to declare victory in this instance, the fact remains that a cure was still unavailable and the lives of these kids remained at risk.

Several of the JDRF representatives had firsthand experience with pioneering technologies and attested that the government's investments were invaluable. They expounded on the health advantages of incorporating the devices and submitted their concordance as embodied evidence for making such machinery more accessible. A number of the delegates took part in clinical trials for CGMs and detailed the positive outcomes of their participation. Volunteers noted that their A1C scores fell drastically while utilizing cutting-edge technologies.[95] As early as 2007, advocates such as McEnery were commenting on the import of the machinery. McEnery explained to the committee, "The CGM gives me freedom, which I did not have before. I no longer worry about having a seizure during the night because my sensor will alert me before this happens. I can participate in sports with ease because I can see what my blood sugar is throughout my games."[96] Still, the refrain of technology not being a cure remained a central component of the message. McEnery continued, "Although the CGM has made my diabetes care much more manageable, it is certainly not a cure. I still have to test my blood sugar twice a day and calculate my insulin doses, and this trial requires that I visit the doctor every two weeks rather than every three months."[97] The organization and its members keep their eyes on the prize, convinced that any distraction from finding a cure endangers lives.

A Promise to Remember

JDRF ambassadors often invoke the phrase "promise to remember me" in their lobbying efforts. They include this when testifying, when writing letters, and when leaving keepsakes with their congresspersons. Youth advocates employ the slogan with the hope that their representatives will recall their struggles when casting votes to fund medical research. It seems to work. Members of Congress frequently parrot the phrase back to the children, assuring them that they will in fact hold their stories close to their hearts. In 2011, Senator Begich told the Children's Congress:

> I will tell you, two years ago, when I first got here, an Alaskan teenager came and visited me to advocate on behalf of the Special Diabetes Program, and she brought me a photo book of her life and what she has been doing to deal with type 1 diabetes, and it was very amazing because you can talk about it, but when you see the photos of her life unfold from day one and as she went through it, it was pretty impactful to me. It is a document and a booklet that I still keep in my office to remind me of the impact and the stories that are all around this issue.[98]

Personal narratives fabricate a direct link to the machinery in Washington, reaffirming that political intimacy can have profound effects. And, to be sure, the JDRF's advocacy efforts have been fruitful in crafting working relationships on Capitol Hill, securing resources, and keeping issues relevant to type 1 diabetes circulating in the public sphere.

The word "promise" is especially fitting in this context. Yes, it emphasizes one's word, but it is also a synonym for "potential." The promise of a cure offers hope in the face of a disease that is otherwise destroying these kids from the inside out.

Framing diabetes as a fatal disease rather than one easily managed is fundamental to understanding the JDRF's discourse. Indeed, should the group emphasize management, its message and motivation for political operatives to act would be emphatically different. Note the influence stressing a cure has on the testimony of Patrick Gould, one of the four siblings from Nashville with type 1 diabetes: "I just want everybody to know that a cure is coming and to hang in there, just hang tight. That is what keeps me going, is that I know that it will be cured eventually and it will be cured soon. So everybody just needs to hang in there and do your best until we do not have to worry about this anymore."[99] A cure is what keeps him vigilant and until it is discovered, worry will permeate his livelihood. At every opportunity, be it an obstinate teenager unwilling to rehearse the routines necessary to survive, a parent worn down by the slog of everyday life, or a scientist making a case for pluripotent stem cell research, the prospect of a cure is dependent on Congress's commitment to remembering them. The pairing of children with fatalistic consequences if action is not taken fashions a sympathetic, commanding, and ultimately persuasive message. Still, a striking paradox stems from this corporeal activism. The very presence of the children seems to prevent fatalism from overtaking the rhetoric completely. That is, far from being entirely overrun by despair, the JDRF's embodied overtures spur movement, ambition, and hope. Witnesses to the JDRF's struggles intervene actively on their behalf, not being entangled in remorse but inspired by the young advocates.

The JDRF continues to build from its achievements and adapt its agenda to confront the many challenges that accompany diabetes's evolving public character. In 2012, the JDRF stripped itself of the name "Juvenile Diabetes Research Foundation," adopting only the acronym, to reflect the fact that most people with type 1 diabetes are not children. That, coupled with the desire to secure additional Medicare funds for CGMs, led the organization to testify before the Senate's Special Aging Committee in 2013, even as it continued to use child activists. Senator Ben Nelson opened the hearing by saying, "Type 1 diabetes is no longer a juvenile disease . . . In fact, 85 percent of people in the US living with type 1 diabetes are adults."[100] Going further, he pointed out that, "diabetes is the leading cause of end-stage renal disease (ESRD), which cost Medicare $29 billion in 2009."[101] Here the ominous presence of death brings together the lives of people with diabetes and the economic security of the nation. The development of technologies such as the artificial pancreas are vital not only for those living in the present but also because such technologies will inevitably influence the economic well-being of Medicare.

The placement of child advocates in a forum traditionally dedicated to the nation's senior citizens raises questions about the reception of their testimony in Congress, especially since the majority of older people diagnosed with diabetes have type 2. The JDRF rarely engaged type 2 diabetes overtly in its previous lobbying efforts, and the articulation to that disease, while potentially fruitful, could have significant effects on its campaigns. Over the years, type 2 diabetes was mentioned occasionally by the Children's Congress, but almost always with the caveat that type 1 could not be controlled as easily. Nelson, for example, teased out these differences by saying, "unlike sufferers of type 2 diabetes which we know can sometimes be reversed with lifestyle changes, individuals with type 1 diabetes are often diagnosed early, without a cure, and left insulin-dependent for life."[102] Professional basketball player Ray Allen, who was advocating on behalf of his young son, told the Senate:

> It isn't Walker's fault that he has type 1 diabetes. There's nothing he or we did to cause it. It isn't diet or lifestyle related, as is the case with type 2 diabetes. Genetics are part of it but there is no history of type 1 diabetes in our family. We do know this: Type 1 diabetes is an autoimmune disease. The body launches an attack on the cells that produce insulin, eventually destroying them and leaving people with type 1 diabetes dependent on synthetic insulin to survive. But insulin is not a cure.[103]

The refrain that medicine is a poor substitute for a life free of chronic illness is revived here but delivered seconds after the suggestion that diet and lifestyle changes could easily alter type 2 diabetes. Framing the more common form of diabetes with subtle contempt, as suggested in both of the above comments, can have multiple effects depending on the publics that receive them. It could stunt identification with a sizable population and foreclose possible affinity politics that would be expedient on Capitol Hill. Far from only functioning as a divisive rhetoric, however, the circulation of such messages could strike back at those living with type 1. The guilt and blame that tend to haunt those with type 2 does, in many ways, get tethered to people with type 1 diabetes as they age. The projection of the sovereign subject is not easily marginalized in scripts about diabetes, and great care must be taken to ensure it does not reproduce itself on various bodies that struggle with glucose irregularities.

The JDRF continues its work of educating the public about type 1 diabetes. Even as the children adopt an ambivalent approach to management, they advocate incessantly for a cure. They do the important work of bringing visibility to the multitude of problems underlying the lives of people like them. They are steady with their focus on a cure and unapologetically brazen in their approach, continually refocusing their aspirations to meet the challenges of the day. They command the attention of presidents, of Congress, and even members of the US Supreme Court, such as Sonia Sotomayor. She is, after all, one of them. Justice Sotomayor and the transcendent rhetoric that surrounded her confirmation is the focus of the next chapter.

4

Containing Sotomayor

Narratives of Personal Restraint

When President Barack Obama announced Sonia Sotomayor as his choice to succeed Justice David Souter on the nation's highest court, reactions from his political opposition were swift, vehement, and vicious. Critics assailed Sotomayor as "dumb," a "bully," and an intellectual lightweight who could not hold her own against conservative judicial icon Antonin Scalia.[1] Political operatives defending her nomination retorted that she graduated summa cum laude from Princeton, was a confident litigator, and possessed more experience on the appeals circuit than any person ever appointed to the US Supreme Court. Sotomayor's detractors and supporters disagreed most explicitly when engaging the influence her Latina identity would have on judicial rulings. Whereas some argued her life experiences offered a unique perspective for rendering decisions, others feared an inherent bias on issues such as affirmative action and immigration. Pundits latched onto an address Sotomayor had delivered in which she stated, "I would hope that a wise Latina woman with the richness of her experiences would more often than not reach a better conclusion than a white male who hasn't lived that life." That rumination was an allusion to remarks made by Sandra Day O'Connor about the incongruities of gender representation in the judicial sphere. Sotomayor's speech likewise attempted to highlight inequalities by giving presence to the complicated features of Latina identities, the necessity of resisting a universal understanding of wisdom, and the circumscribed roles of women and minorities (not to mention those who live at the intersection of these subject positions) in the legal system.[2] Despite the provocative and nuanced themes laid out in that speech, Sotomayor's opponents charged her with being a reverse racist who would create policy via empathy rather than originalist interpretive schemas. When Alabama Senator Jeff Sessions commented that Sotomayor would shape the court "in a way that would be different from our heritage so far," he was making no secret about whose heritage he believed was under attack.³ Sotomayor was positioned as erratic, petulant, and threatening in a legal sphere that prizes decorous banter and judicial restraint.⁴

The Obama administration responded to these racially charged allegations by presenting Sotomayor's lifetime of managing type 1 diabetes to evidence her deliberate temperament and personal fortitude. Decades of managing diabetes provided compelling anecdotal evidence that Sotomayor had the wherewithal to navigate the quotidian complexities of a notoriously vicious disease and, by extension, the demands of the job. Diabetes management became a politically expedient way to display an embodiment of judicial prudence, performatively constituting a measured character befitting a Supreme Court justice. Media outlets published assurances from Sotomayor's physician that attested to her discipline. *Time* magazine reported, "According to her doctor, she has excellent control of her diabetes, with consistent blood sugars better than 98% of diabetics. Her hemoglobin A1C levels, the best measure of diabetes control, have consistently been less than 6.5 percent, the optimal level as defined by all diabetes organizations. She has no evidence of any complications of diabetes or even any early signs that they may develop."⁵ The statistical claims made by the doctor are speculative, if not hyperbolic, as diabetes is an individuated disease marked by varying routines and goals not easily reducible to comparative analysis stemming from aggregate data.⁶ The doctor's narrative was especially remarkable next to biographical details of Sotomayor's life that customarily indicate obstacles to good health, including that she was raised by a single mother in a low-income part of the Bronx. Against all odds, from the economic barriers that tend to hasten the demise of people with diabetes or the institutional impediments that portend a lifetime of complications, Sotomayor had transcended the limits of her disease. As a result, her story materialized as an American dream narrative that accentuated personal responsibility and hard work.

The White House decision to emphasize Sotomayor's diabetes as a reflection of her tenacity and unmitigated success was foundational to establishing a priming device for her performance at the confirmation hearings. Scholars such as José Esteban Muñoz and Linda Martín Alcoff have observed that Sotomayor's performance before the Senate was akin to an exercise in passing that was recognizable to people of color who find themselves in the crosshairs of racial animus.[7] Reserved and contemplative throughout the event, Sotomayor occupied a tenuous space familiar to members of marginalized groups. I argue that attention to Sotomayor's diabetes in the weeks leading up to the confirmation was a co-constitutive element of this performative constraint, not resting apart from her Latina identity but instead being essential to the cultivation of her judicial persona. Lisa Flores has noted that the discursive circulation of raced bodies frequently signals an "excessive and chaotic" entity.[8] Institutions justify their disciplinary tendencies by casting people of color as inherently exotic and threatening, enacting punitive measures in the name of the nation to reproduce racial hierarchies. The invocation of Sotomayor's diabetes mitigated these predictable rhetorical tropes, accentuating her character as moderate and affable, not intemperate and ungovernable. Sotomayor's condition ultimately framed her, in the words of Josue David Cisneros, as a "reasonable and objective citizen-subject."[9]

This chapter privileges the idea that diabetes is a disability, not only because it falls under the legal definition as outlined by the Americans with Disabilities Act (ADA), but also because diabetes is made culturally intelligible as an aberration of normative health accompanied by a litany of medical repercussions and burdensome maintenance practices. To be sure, diabetes is like many disabilities in that it is often "invisible within the immediate temporal frame."[10] The consequences of diabetes generally become recognizable only during emergencies, such as the debilitating effects of hypoglycemia, or through physical markers such as amputation. Even as many people with diabetes have learned to manage the disease, most are also captive to a recitation of painful routines, such as finger pricks and shots, that demand unending self-surveillance.[11] Personal control is closely aligned with positive values, "described as a marker of virtue, will, maturity, and autonomy; declining to control it indicated laziness, gluttony, or, simply, ignorance."[12] In short, the discipline exhibited by people with diabetes is linked directly to judgments others make about their character, personal conviction, and productivity.

In what follows, I give primacy to disability as a vital component of intersectional critique to illustrate how incorporeal abstractions such as "wisdom" and "restraint" materialize heterogeneously, not univocally, through rhetorical practices in situ. I contemplate how discourses ordinarily thought to regulate individual bodily performances also govern cultural narratives about judgment and the institutional hierarchies that shape expectations and representations about those positioned on the outskirts of power structures. Centralizing considerations of disabled bodies in research, Lisa Duggan has argued, "is not a call to add disability to an intersectional matrix of race, gender, class, sexuality, nationality, religion. It is a call to step aside, provisionally, to imagine theory and politics from the capacious 'standpoint' of disability."[13] Privileging disabilities encourages critics to think differently about the materiality of bodies in particular contexts—in this instance the politics underwriting the judicial sphere—even as disability can never be compartmentalized from other social formations such as race and gender. Sotomayor's Latina heritage was deemed a threat to the fictionalized legal objectivity constituting the judiciary, which has historically been composed of white men who have assuredly never been objective in their judicial orientations. The introduction of Sotomayor's diabetes instigated an alternative narrative to the accusations made by conservatives about her status as a "wise Latina," underscoring her prudence to assure detractors that she would not subvert the normative workings of the judiciary.

Even as word of Sotomayor's diabetes circulated extensively in the days before the Senate met, it disappeared almost completely during the hearings. The ephemeral nature of chronic disease in this context—it is literally rendered invisible—seemingly took hold, acting as a backdrop to the unfolding political drama. This sudden evacuation of disease suggests one instance when a chronic condition acted first as a structuring mechanism for interpreting her character and then as a paradiscourse for attitudinizing her persona as circumspect. Throughout this saga, Sotomayor's resolve was brought to life as a prudential skill, one that was encapsulated by management's conceptual plasticity: She could be depicted as deliberately focused on her health but also casual about her diabetes. To cement claims made throughout the chapter, I also look past the hearings to briefly examine Sotomayor's memoir *My Beloved World*, where diabetes bookends the text. I explore how the reintroduction of diabetes recuperates and nuances her complicated identity by returning to themes accentuated prior to the hearings. Diabetes in both the hearings and the memoir occupies the margins and I bring it center stage to investigate its shifting rhetorical functions.

This chapter acts as the basis for elucidating a third heuristic to contemplate diabetes management: that of personal fortitude and transcendence. The sovereign subject who overcomes disease and illness through the sheer force of personal will and dogged determination surfaces time and again in popular culture, often being captured by phrases such as "super crip" or "inspiration porn." These fantastical narratives centered on individuals who defy seemingly insurmountable obstacles (be they bodily or culturally imposed) are ubiquitous in stories about illness, disease, and disability. The miraculous practices of these characters are a recurring feature of news reports, industry magazines, and the mythos of solitary tenacity. And while it would be careless to suggest that there are no narratives of success and perseverance in diabetes history, it is also the case that such revelatory figures often eclipse institutional failures, structural ills, and systemic solutions for grappling with diabetes. In the case of Sotomayor, such typifications also disregard the intricate vestiges of identity, politics, and treatment that configure life with diabetes. The intersection of disability, gender, race, and class essential to the justice's life story offers compelling lessons about the precarity of marginalized groups, the rhetoric of self-surveillance, and the staying power of empowerment narratives.

Disability and Productive Intersectional Critique

Social constructions of race, gender, and disability have been mutually informative for much of America's history. From the bodies made disabled by slave owners to eugenic movements that situated racial minorities as "feeble-minded," the intersecting vectors of disability, race, and gender have long been publicly conjoined and usually to the detriment of people of color.[14] Despite (or perhaps because of) this legacy, there has been a discernable absence of people with disabilities in historical accounts of noteworthy people of color.[15] Of course, disabilities exist on a broad spectrum, ranging from physical immobility to somatic conditions. The possible articulations among race, gender, and disability are limitless and their coterminous relationships are culturally pervasive, if often unrecognized. In order to centralize considerations of intersectional identity, many researchers have begun using disability critical race theory (DisCrit), while others in the humanities have devised so-called cripistemologies, to elucidate historical ills and bring attention to the unique challenges facing people of color who have disabilities.[16] These novel approaches for contemplating intersectional identities attempt to correct genealogies that marginalize, misrepresent, and misunderstand the ways gender, race, and disability manifest in tandem.

Perspectives that privilege the mutual constitution of disability, race, and gender follow an extensive corpus of intersectional work that seeks to make visible marginalized subject positions and offer insight into the multifarious nature of identity. Karma Chávez and Cindy Griffin argue that intersectional critique enables the creation of frameworks that give presence to "complex facets of identity and subjectivity" critical to investigating the materialization of power and privilege among non-normative people.[17] They promote a "conceptual messiness" that redirects attention away from normative scripts of being and toward those that interrupt taken-for-granted features of cultural belonging.[18] Intersectional critique delineates how subjects are produced and recognized, troubling simplistic notions of interpellation and the formation of personhood. Sara McKinnon has suggested that an intersectional approach to criticism is especially imperative when essentialist rhetorics steer public transcripts because they help to illuminate and challenge "whose voices, bodies, and experiences should have access to material and discursive space in the public."[19] Those who occupy the margins are often perceived as threats to institutions such as the judicial sphere and its attributes of narrative rationality, good speech, and embodied affect.[20]

Intersectionality is more than an amalgamation of categories that can be easily atomized based on previously held understandings about race, disability, and gender.[21] Rather than imagining static categories that engage unending invocations of identity, intersectional critique might best be thought of as a rhetorical style, a constitutive mode of signification that calls attention to the effects of discourse as contingent and contextual, both fungible over time and illustrative in its situated materialization.[22] Leslie Hahner persuasively argues that intersectionality is best conceived as the "juncture through which rhetorical forms value particular identifications and performances."[23] This approach "designates the symbolic, material, and affective connections through which a subject engages a particular discourse."[24] Hahner promotes a provisional modality of intersectionality, one that draws attention to the mobility of identification and the rhetorical forms that actualizes some identities and inhibits others. Critics who bring into focus different constellations of identification can yield novel insights about the intersectional nature of identity and thereby expand the possibilities of intersectional criticism.

Centralizing intersectionality in discussions of health resists the institutional tendency to compartmentalize markers such as gender, disability, and race and also interrupts understandings of medical phenomena as "natural" outcomes of particular identities. Illness and disease are products of cultural articulation just as much as they are biomedical realities. Diseases such as sickle-cell anemia and Tay-Sachs, for instance, have both been wedded to racial categories, even as scholars such as Troy Duster have shown these connections are social outcomes and not foundationally genetic.[25] Depression is not simply an effect of the body, but an array of affective states that are initiated by factors as disparate as racism and socioeconomic status. Diabetes is no exception to this cultural engineering. The condition is often made intelligible through simplistic scripts about race and age rather than considerations of class and geography, and almost always in ways that eclipse diabetes's complicated etiological origins. People with type 2 diabetes, for example, are frequently imagined as people of color, not only in medico-scientific literature about genetics but also in media narratives depicting the disease.[26] These oversimplifications have the effect of constituting diabetes in circumscribed ways, hindering nuanced investigations of its conceptual contours.

To give just one example, Latina theorist Gloria Anzaldúa, perhaps the most widely cited Latina scholar of our time, lived with diabetes. In writings about her life, however, it is commonly and incorrected assumed that she had type 2. Like Sotomayor, Anzaldúa actually lived with type 1.[27] The racialization of the condition, along with the fact that Anzaldúa was diagnosed later in life, leads many people to make false assumptions about the manifestation of her diabetes and the impact it had on her work. What does it mean to articulate Anzaldúa's identity to type 2 diabetes, a disease underlined by projections of guilt and excessiveness, rather than type 1, an autoimmune disease that attacks the body mysteriously and with little notice? I do not mean to reinforce the shaming that haunts people with type 2 diabetes, and in fact I find such impulses deplorable. Still, the rhetorical consequences of a scholar and activist known widely for her "border crossing" being constituted by one disease, and not the other, produces divergent interpretive schemas for contemplating how Anzaldúa and her scholarship are understood. As the following analysis shows, in a culture that prizes hard work and discipline it is not simply diabetes that is racialized—control and good judgment are as well.

Sotomayor's ascent to the US Supreme Court transpired in a politico-judicial sphere that has long been hostile to women, minorities, and people with disabilities.[28] Abstractions such as "wisdom" have been guarded by so-called rational actors who embody a prudence that typically has been consecrated through the bodies of white men. Rhetorically, Sotomayor's diabetes materializes ideas such as restraint and control, allowing those supporting her nomination to move her into the space of judicial power. It is not simply that Sotomayor was a model minority who lived the American Dream. Rather, rhetorics of managerial perseverance imparted a medicinal prudence onto Sotomayor that could be translated positively in the judicial sphere.

Courting Sotomayor

In the weeks prior to Sotomayor's nomination and following the announcement of her candidacy, ample narratives surfaced about her easily excitable persona. From the furor over the "wise Latina" speech to various media reports about her seething character, Sotomayor was portrayed as a person whose emotions overruled her ability to administer justice in a collegial and even-handed manner. These reports tended to accentuate diversity as a social burden and not a benefit, difference as a barrier to be overcome, and the inassimilable qualities of cultural pride.[29] Among the most egregious of these appraisals was that published by the *New Republic*'s Jeffrey Rosen, a profile that smacks of racial caricature and sexist innuendo. Rosen's piece is heavy on biographical details and encumbered by professional gossip.[30] He opens the column with snapshots of Sotomayor's life (and not her qualifications), dramatizing her "compelling" story by including her humble upbringing and the diabetes that she has lived with since age eight. Reporters frequently use the personal histories of public servants to open features and whet the appetites of readers. This stylistic choice was common when Sotomayor was being introduced to audiences and was not unique to Rosen. However, the

New Republic placed these details below a headline that read: "The Case Against Sotomayor: Indictments of Obama's Front Runner to Replace Souter," imposing a lens that explicitly merges her personality and her judicial philosophy. Of course, the press has a disquieting and sexist habit of using personal stories to humanize women in the public eye and often with the effect of conflating personal and professional personas into one. This column is no exception. The opening paragraph also explicitly draws attention to race, noting Sotomayor's Puerto Rican heritage, that she would be the first "Hispanic" on the Court, and that a logical second choice would have been Ken Salazar, then Secretary of the Interior. Rosen expands on biographical details using anonymous sources, including a former clerk who said that Sotomayor "grew up in a situation of disadvantage, and was able, by virtue of the system operating in such a fair way, to accomplish what she did. I think she sees the law as an instrument that can accomplish the same thing for other people, a system that, if administered fairly, can give everyone the fair break they deserve, regardless of who they are." In this mnemoscape, the personal is explicitly merged with the political and through a language that has traditionally rankled the chains of conservatives. The administering of "fairness" is certainly a euphemism for affirmative action, but even cast in a positive light such framing functions oddly as a form of telepathy for reading Sotomayor's raison d'être.

Rosen quotes sources who express "questions about her temperament" and "her judicial craftsmanship," because Sotomayor is seemingly not "a judicial star of the highest intellectual caliber." He relays the feelings of yet another unnamed source who argues, "She has an inflated opinion of herself, and is domineering during oral arguments, but her questions aren't penetrating and don't get to the heart of the issue." Although Rosen never explicitly connects race and gender to these criticisms, the form of his essay adopts a deductive logic underscored by considerations of both. There is an operative enthymeme that bridges her background, indeed her identity, with her supposed shortcomings. Perhaps most unsettling is that Rosen admits that he has not "read enough of Sotomayor's opinions to have a confident sense of them," nor had he "talked to enough of Sotomayor's detractors and supporters, to get a fully balanced picture of her strengths." Ta-Nehisi Coates rightly retorted, "I can't get past that line—mostly because . . . Rosen is attacking Sotomayor's ability to do the necessary intellectual heavy-lifting, while explicitly neglecting to do any of his own."[31] Despite rejoinders to such reporting, remarks such as Rosen's were omnipresent in the press. Journalists conveyed that Sotomayor "can be demanding and exacting" and that she had been accused of being too "outspoken and temperamental on the bench."[32] Time and again media talking heads returned to the image of a fiery Latina whose disruptive personality would not suit the national interest.

Initially Sotomayor's diabetes was similarly articulated as a burdensome feature of her personality. Even before she was recommended by Obama, there was much speculation that living with diabetes might prevent her from consideration for the bench. Appointments to the Court are characterized by long tenures, often with the nomination of a person in early middle age who might have decades left to serve. Health complications trouble these protracted tenures, making Sotomayor's diabetes a potential stumbling block. CNN's Jeffrey Toobin argued, "It would be irresponsible for any president not to make the health of the nominee a major subject of concern, because presidents want decades of service from their nominees."[33] Supreme Court scholar Howard Ball, himself a person with type 2 diabetes, surmised that Sotomayor had likely developed a strict regimen for managing her diabetes, but still believed she would not become a "viable option" for the administration.[34]

Ball can hardly be ridiculed for his prediction, which is otherwise supported by historical evidence. The legacy of the Supreme Court is replete with examples of health crises that have heralded a warning to presidents contemplating judicial replacements.[35] Justice Horace Lurton, nominated to the bench by William Taft in 1909, has become a cautionary tale. He was appointed at the age of sixty-five and died just four years later. Dwight Eisenhower's selection of Charles Whittaker lives in infamy because that judge had a nervous breakdown while serving on the job.[36] It is believed that Bill Clinton wanted to appoint Richard Arnold to the bench but could not because cancerous tumors reemerged in his body years after being treated for lymphoma.[37] Of course, health complications need not disqualify competent jurists from serving. Both Sandra Day O'Connor and Ruth Bader Ginsburg publicly battled cancer during their incumbencies. John Roberts has long been rumored to have epilepsy, but if true, it has never been confirmed in the press. Conspiracy theorists on the right have gone as far as accusing Roberts of upholding the individual mandate of the Affordable Care Act because of this ailment, and lack of corroboration by the press only fuels such speculation.

Sotomayor's cautious transparency about her diabetes had the potential to further a narrative that stressed a body out of bounds, one that articulated a lack of control over her health as indexing something more fundamental about her character. Because diabetes is frequently imagined as a sign of excess and decline, especially when articulated to a racialized body, it is not surprising that media reports often emphasized plight and precarity when scrutinizing her health.[38] Outlets including National Public Radio repeated the statistic that people with diabetes generally live seven to ten years less than those without it, even as they reported the disease is more manageable than ever before.[39] Discussions of Sotomayor's health inevitably produced questions about her longevity and what her regimens revealed about her personality. CNN, for example, explicitly connected the control of blood sugars to moral fortitude. Keep in mind that the normative glucose reading for a person without diabetes is 90 and that number is the goalpost against which people with diabetes are often measured in the public eye. CNN quoted an endocrinologist who discussed typical A1C scores for people in Sotomayor's socioeconomic class, noting that she should score 7–8 percent, which translates to an average reading of 154 on the low end of that scale and a 183 on the high end. He remarked that if the result came back at 13 percent, "you'd say how responsible is this person?"[40] Another endocrinologist interviewed in that same story countered, saying he would want to see her A1C below 5 percent, which is an average of 97 and virtually impossible for a person with type 1 diabetes to achieve. Despite diabetes's recalcitrant effects, political columnist Sam Stein observed correctly that a "history of coronary disease, high blood pressure, [or] Crohn's disease . . . can present far more difficult medical quandaries."[41]

The preoccupation with control surfaced repeatedly in the reporting and often in close association with diabetes. One doctor told the *New York Times* that "the public had a right to know how the judge was controlling her diabetes—and how well."[42] That may be true, but the transference from medical condition to personality in much of the coverage was striking. One media outlet commented that to "dispense with any health concerns about Judge Sotomayor, officials said the White House contacted her doctor and independent experts to determine whether diabetes, which she learned she had at eight years old, might be problematic and concluded it would not. The Obama team also interviewed colleagues on the Second Circuit to check out reports that she was difficult to get along with, and was reassured it was not true."[43] I pause here to emphasize the close interrelationship between the unmanaged associations with diabetes and the degree to which control over the disease was made proxemic to incivility. There is a metonymic slide from one to the other in diabetes discourse, and in this report a positive association with disease is made intelligible next to potential deficiencies of character.

The intense focus on control took a sharp turn when diabetes pivoted from being a potential health disadvantage to a condition that trumpeted Sotomayor's qualifications to be confirmed. Almost overnight, media outlets relayed that the justice had persevered through life's hardships despite the hand she had been dealt. Life with a chronic disease presented not only obstacles, but opportunities; not just the trappings of management but proof that she could transcend the condition. Sotomayor's advocates transformed the ubiquitous roadblocks presented by diabetes into evidence of her prudence and personal restraint, giving presence to a wisdom befitting a Supreme Court justice. The statement from Sotomayor's physician mentioned at the start of this chapter, the one that contended she controlled her blood sugars better than 98 percent of people with diabetes, resonated with a "humble beginnings" American dream mythos and offered an alternative narrative for the approaching hearings.

The reassurances from Sotomayor's physician that she had not developed any eye, kidney, or nerve complications due to diabetes had immediate effect. The news that Sotomayor managed her health vigilantly supplanted her once-out-of-control excessiveness with tales of constraint and thoughtfulness. The *New York Daily News* told readers that she was "very casual about [her diabetes]. It's not something that's held her back in any way."[44] Sotomayor's diabetes was framed as a catalyst for success and motivated her many accomplishments. *New York Times* reporter Sheryl Gay Stolberg contended that "Ms. Sotomayor's lifelong struggle with diabetes lent a sense of urgency." Stolberg quotes an acquaintance who recalls, "It made her think, 'I'm not going to be around forever, I have to keep moving.'"[45] One of Sotomayor's friends remembered, "Sonia told me many years ago that because of her diabetes, she had only a certain amount of time to live . . . She's lived maybe 20 years longer than she ever thought she would."[46] A former colleague conveyed, "She was very tenacious . . . We would be in a tense interview with a candidate and she would be shooting herself with insulin in the back of the hand."[47] Still another asserted, "She'll be eating Chinese dumplings . . . and she'll say, 'Excuse me sweetie,' and pull out the kit and inject her insulin."[48] Rather than presenting challenges to a long tenure on the court, diabetes is articulated with tropes emphasizing self-determination and intuitive management, a common sense that would be invaluable in the third branch of government. The public is left to deduce that type 1 diabetes is inherent to her no-nonsense attitude and the attention to detail that characterizes her legal opinions. In short, control was now emblematic of her personality and judicial philosophy, which earlier had been merged negatively as intemperate and in a racially charged manner. Astute readers will note that the trope of management facilitated and reconciled a number of seemingly disparate impulses about diabetes care that suggest prudential action: She acted both casually and with a sense of urgency, deliberately but with the spontaneity required by a life with diabetes.

Refrains about Sotomayor's diabetes in the press were structured by discourses of moderation, balance, and thoughtfulness. Numerous articles that featured diabetes as a part of her life's story also extolled Sotomayor's moderate judicial philosophy. The *Times* article that pivoted on the trope of "urgency" mentioned above, for example, magnified her cautious political leanings. "Ms. Sotomayor's political persona hewed carefully to the contours of New York, liberal but not particularly ideological. And, unusual in a city where Democrats outnumber Republicans five to one, she registered as an independent." The *Washington Post* opined that diabetes was among her "frailties" but situated it in the context of her living an "understated" life and as a person hesitant to subscribe to politically extreme positions.[49] The *Post* contended that as a student at Princeton, Sotomayor was "active in Latino student affairs but not a bomb thrower." This stunning assessment of Latino activism exacerbates the racial stereotypes underlying segments of the reporting, even as diabetes is placed close by to accentuate her constraint.[50] Indeed, one news outlet reported that Latinos were skeptical of her nomination, wondering if she would be too centrist on the bench.[51] Repeatedly, her diagnosis was located in proximity to her "moderate judicial record." The repetitious theme of a woman of color too passionate and empathetic for the court was tempered by discourses of restraint that regularly featured diabetes.

Perhaps the most explicit joining of health and restraint came in early July 2009 when it was revealed that Sotomayor had recused herself from a case because one of the claimants lived with diabetes. The article outlined a 1997 case in which Sotomayor claimed to have "personal knowledge regarding the claims."[52] Although the justice indicated she could not remember why she recused herself from *John Doe v. City of New York*, the reporter surmised her chronic condition was the likely reason. The plaintiff on the suit had diabetes and claimed he had been denied medication by the Department of Correction, leading to pain and complications. The city later settled with him. One scholar argued that if Sotomayor's diabetes was the deciding factor for recusal, it was an "exceptionally cautious" choice. This contemplativeness was reflected in a letter Sotomayor sent to the Senate judicial committee in which she stated, "I have chosen to recuse myself from cases, even when not technically required by ethical rules."[53] Within the span of a month, diabetes went from a vicious condition that might inhibit service to one that reflected her measured demeanor and stoic impartiality.

Media accounts of Sotomayor's life with diabetes both interrupted and reinforced traditional scripts of disability and the requisite accompaniments of hard work and focused control. The degree of agency media outlets attributed to Sotomayor suggests both a hegemonic ableism that reassures able-bodied audiences that this disability is not so bad but also provides an opportunity to resist racist and sexist discourse that paints people of color (with disabilities) as unmanageable. Sotomayor's advocates may have represented her life with diabetes narrowly but did so in a way that, perhaps inadvertently, laid the groundwork for conversations about the productive nature of her identity. Tobin Siebers contends that disability often functions as a masquerade, refiguring the "critical frameworks for identifying and questioning the complicated ideologies on which social injustice and oppression depend."[54] Disabilities can be exaggerated, downplayed, or strategically deployed to subvert the normative workings of the political sphere. In this context, Sotomayor's diabetes may have reinforced notions of management that actualize scripts of individual transcendence and discipline but nonetheless made prejudices about people with diabetes work in her favor.

To summarize, diabetes first materialized as an extension of Sotomayor's supposedly excessive and chaotic body. Then it signified a containment mechanism that represented constraint and transcendence. In looking to this pattern, I am not asserting that Sotomayor's diabetes erased discussions of her race and gender. It certainly did not. Conservative critics continued to assail her relentlessly, even after it became apparent that she would be confirmed. Rather, the use of diabetes to illustrate control and discipline appeared to be strategically employed by the Obama administration, just as elements of her appearance at the confirmation hearings were monitored to downplay her ethnicity.[55] Although the administration could not control the ways the press relayed Sotomayor's diabetes to the public, I argue the effects of this discourse functioned as a priming device for interpreting her personal resolve. In the following section I examine Sotomayor's performance at the hearings to explore the materialization of an incorporeal concept—judicial restraint—on a body rife with symbolic import. The confirmation actualized Sotomayor's tenacity and prudential disposition, highlighting her contemplative persona in the face of a hostile congressional committee.

Confirmation Bias

Sotomayor's confirmation hearings divulged how abstract notions such as "restraint" and "wisdom" are institutionally monitored to reconstitute universal performances of prudence in the judicial sphere. In many ways, the hearings were characterized by the typical banter that occurs between judicial nominees and Senate committee members, with the most explosive emanating from Republicans, who displayed fiery rebukes and toxic iterations of whiteness.[56] These exchanges generated a wealth of scholarship about the political, structural, and representational stakes undergirding the appointment of a woman of color to the bench. Scholars used the event to examine everything from the impact of women's interest groups on the process to the history of pro-immigration rulings among Supreme Court justices.[57] Some scrutinized her nomination to gauge the heterogeneity of political investments among Latinos, while others dissected the accusations that Sotomayor was intellectually inferior to past nominees. For the record—she is not.[58] Attention to Sotomayor's diabetes further explains how her decorous persona emerged through invocations of restraint that materialized as a form of judiciousness sanctioned in the American legal system.

Publicity about Sotomayor's diabetes stopped circulating almost completely during the week she was being vetted by Congress. Her critics were not able to impede her nomination by focusing on diabetes and thus moved on to more opportunistic castigations after news about her chronic condition reached its saturation point. The repackaging of her medical condition as a strength and not a weakness left her opposition with little ammunition on this front, so they focused their energies on controversies that had already garnered media coverage, such as her past speeches. In fact, in a process that spanned four full days, her diabetes was mentioned just twice, once by Senator Dick Durbin and once by an old friend from high school. Following the narrative that developed late in the press coverage, Durbin revisited the association between her condition and her biography. He opined:

> Judge Sotomayor, you have overcome many obstacles in your life that have given you an understanding of the daily realities and struggles faced by everyday people. You grew up in a housing complex in the Bronx. You overcame a diagnosis of juvenile diabetes at age 8 and the death of your father at age 9. Your mother worked two jobs so she could afford to send you and your brothers to Catholic schools, and you earned scholarships to Princeton and Yale.[59]

Her friend, Columbia law professor Theodore Shaw, followed suit, remembering: "Sonia did not live a life of privilege. She lost her father at a very young age. She had been diagnosed with diabetes even before she came to high school. It was not something I remember her talking about. She simply carried herself with an air of dignity, seriousness, of purpose, and a sense that she was going somewhere."[60] This characterization reiterated what had become common sense among the political elite: that Sotomayor's diabetes was largely a non-issue and, if anything, accentuated her determination, control, and fortitude.

Even as audiences were primed to read Sotomayor's persona as restrained, Senate Republicans threw to the wind any notion that they should do the same. The asymmetrical performances of power are particularly striking when one considers that Sotomayor was compelled to perform diffidently even as the white men interrogating her did not. The confirmation hearing was awash in racist remarks, both implicit and explicit, that make Sotomayor's performance especially praiseworthy. Time and again senators made incendiary statements and the magistrate would deflect them with understated gusto. Knowing that Sotomayor was a prosecutor at home in combative settings helps to explain, in part, her requiescence. A lifetime of navigating sexism and racism offers equal enlightenment. Senator Tom Colburn of Oklahoma channeled Ricky Ricardo during the event, saying, "You'll have a lot of 'splainin' to do."[61] Senator Lindsey Graham of South Carolina told her she would be confirmed unless she had a "meltdown," and repeatedly returned to accusations that she was "temperamental," "aggressive," "excitable," and "angry."[62] Latching on to the idea that she ruled by empathy, Senator Jon Kyl of Arizona asked if she has "always been able to find a legal basis for every decision that [she has] rendered as a judge."[63] Multiple senators assured her they were not voting against her because she was Latina, as they would have gladly confirmed Miguel Estrada, a conservative Honduran American Bush appointee with no judicial experience.[64]

Representatives who made particularly egregious remarks shared one common denominator: concern about Sotomayor's legal treatment of issues such as affirmative action and immigration, both of which tend to excite their base and drive fund-raising efforts. As noted earlier, Sotomayor's critics worried she would be sympathetic to race-based discrimination cases, even as law professor Tom Goldstein remarked in the *New York Times* that her judicial record did not reflect such leanings. Sotomayor was part of a three-member appellate court that heard roughly one hundred race-based cases but upheld only ten of them. Nine of those ten decisions were unanimous.[65] This is to say nothing of a right-leaning organization that accused her of fronting a terrorist organization, which turned out to be the Puerto Rican Legal Defense and Education Fund.[66] Rush Limbaugh announced that he was going to buy her a vacuum so that she could clean after her meetings with Belizean Grove, an invitation-only organization composed of powerful women.

The theatrics that structure contemporary Supreme Court confirmations are generally rehearsed well in advance, with few precipitous events occurring during the hearings. It would be surprising if any of the senators participating in the event had not already committed to voting for or against Sotomayor prior to their arrival. As Trevor Parry-Giles writes, "Increased partisan polarization and an amplified sense of the judiciary's political and social importance have magnified the stakes of judicial nominations and created an environment in which presidential administrations avoid deliberation, to seek confirmation at any and all costs."[67] These sentiments seem especially useful in a contemporary context in which a presidential nominee cannot even receive a hearing before an oppositional Senate. Even if she or he did, the public has become primed for the fights that stem from confirmations. In Sotomayor's case, the racial animus directed at her was repugnant but not entirely surprising when considering the tribalism that marks Senate factions.

Although diabetes was rarely mentioned during the hearings, journalistic assessments of Sotomayor's control and moderation resonated when lawmakers repeatedly venerated the concept of judicial restraint. To be clear, I am not asserting a direct correlation between media reports about discipline and questions posed to Sotomayor by individual senators. Rather, the presence given to Sotomayor's diabetes in the weeks leading up to the hearings is essential to interpreting those portions of the transcript that dealt with constitutional impartiality. Sotomayor's character was "constituted by power relations that are far from transparent" and intersectionality's productive complexities, including maintaining a connection among disability, gender, and race, elucidates the creation and reiteration of hierarchical power systems that demanded a circumspect performance during the vetting process.[68]

Numerous senators, including John Cornyn, Chuck Grassley, Diane Feinstein, Al Franken, Patrick Leahy, and Sheldon Whitehouse, all raised the fleeting and undefined notion of judicial restraint. Sotomayor's political opponents wielded the shibboleth to indict her alleged antagonistic disposition. Her supporters, conversely, embraced the accepted characterization that she was deliberate and measured. For example, quoting from a letter written on Sotomayor's behalf, Leahy contended the judge reflects "the type of tempered restraint and moderation necessary for appropriate application of the rule of law" and that she "serves with a moderate voice without displays of bias toward any party based on affiliation, background, sex, color, or religion."[69] Whitehouse concurred, adding, "my Republican colleagues have talked a great deal about judicial modesty and restraint. Fair enough to a point, but that point comes when these words become slogans, not real critiques of your record. Indeed, these calls for restraint and modesty, and complaints about 'activist' judges, are often codewords, seeking a particular kind of judge who will deliver a particular set of political outcomes."[70] After detailing the ways justices such as John Roberts are offered the presumption of objectivity, Whitehouse attested that Sotomayor's "diverse life experience," "broad professional background," and "expertise as a judge at each level of the system" had endowed her with the capacity to make sound judgments.[71] Whitehouse anticipated Muñoz's observation that Sotomayor did not conform to the mythic norms associated with embodied notions of reason. As such, his colleagues across the aisle accused her of rendering decisions on purely affectual grounds, not nominal claims grounded in objectivity.[72]

Sotomayor's overtures toward judicial restraint are especially noteworthy during those parts of the hearing where considerations of gender, race, and health surface in tandem. Graham grilled Sotomayor about her involvement with the Puerto Rican Legal Defense Fund, wanting to know if she advocated for federal funds for abortion while on their board. Sotomayor commented that she was not privy to that organization's legal briefs that advocated for taxpayer funding of abortion but that she did have a hand in other "public health issues." Graham inquired if abortion was, in her opinion, a "public health issue." Sotomayor insisted her thoughts on the matter were irrelevant and deferred to the normative contours of the law. "It wasn't a question of whether I personally viewed it that way or not. The issue was whether the law was settled on what issues the Fund was advocating on behalf of the community it represented."[73] For her, the question became one of making good-faith arguments rooted in the Constitution. The hot-button issue of abortion can only be interpreted through the parameters put into place by the judiciary. The few times disabilities are explicitly mentioned, generally in the context of rulings about the ADA, Sotomayor insisted that courts do not legislate from the bench. Rather, they ensure that Congress works within the parameters of its legislative powers.[74]

Accentuating disability through an intersectional lens makes present features of the testimony that might otherwise remain unnoticed. In one particularly provocative instance from the hearing, which is later revisited in her memoir, Sotomayor touted the necessity of weighing evidence through established legal standards in order to properly adjudicate case law. She recalls a salient moment from her days as a prosecutor when she dismissed charges against a young man who was accused of larceny. The defense lawyer in the case approached Sotomayor and implored her: "I never ever do this, but this kid is innocent. Please look at his background. *He's a kid with a disability.* Talk to his teachers. Look at his life. Look at his record. Here it is."[75] Sotomayor was alarmed by the arrest because the woman who reported the crime never actually saw who stole her pocketbook. Sotomayor recollects: "In that case, she saw a young man that the police had stopped in a subway station with a black jacket and she thought she had seen a black jacket and identified the young man as the one who had stolen her property." Disability is at best as an attribute that positively underscores the man's character and at worst suggests his inability to commit the crime. The anecdote invites the audience to read Sotomayor's empathetic and restrained sensibility that functions well in the occasion: false accusations that are challenged by the constraints of the law and the thoughtfulness of the attending attorneys.

Sotomayor responded to castigations that she was overly empathetic not by dismissing the charges, but by emphasizing fidelity to the law as a form of restraint. In response to a question about experiences guiding judicial philosophy she retorted, "Life experiences have to influence you. We're not robots [who] listen to evidence and don't have feelings. We have to recognize those feelings and put them aside."[76] The point is not to ignore emotion, but to recognize it and practice restraint. In an exchange with Senator Cornyn the following day, she elucidated the effect that different experiences have on judges but that are ultimately checked by the constraints of the legal sphere. She observed, "I think life experiences generally, whether it's that I'm a Latina or was a State prosecutor or have been a commercial litigator or been a trial judge and an appellate judge, that the mixture of all of those things, the amalgam of them, helped me to listen and understand. But all of us understand, because that's the kind of judges we have proven ourselves to be, we rely on the law to command the results in the case."⁷⁷ Judicial emotion here "is to be temporally isolated—that is, experienced only at a predecisional moment—and operationally neutered—that is, disabled from exerting any effects on behavior and decision making."⁷⁸ Remarkably, Senator Chuck Schumer spent ample time engaging Sotomayor about those plaintiffs she felt empathy for, but felt forced to decide against because of the rule of law. This included family members of those killed on TWA flight 800, which crashed off the coast of Long Island in 1996.

Sotomayor's diabetes also receded from view in the press, which is hardly surprising in light of the fact that it was downplayed significantly during her Senate appearance. A search of the terms "Sotomayor" and "diabetes" during the week of the confirmation yielded zero results and "Sotomayor" and "diabetic" produced only seven, several of which were from the same essay reproduced in multiple media outlets. In the few instances that diabetes is alluded to, it is articulated with results that followed the themes that have dominated this chapter. A headline from the *St. Paul Pioneer Press* extolled, "What Has Sotomayor Revealed? Self-Control." That broadsheet relayed that "Physically, too, Sotomayor has held her ground, despite a cast on her right leg and a lifelong diabetic condition . . . Her body language has been commanding."⁷⁹ The attention to Sotomayor's body was incessant, if not peculiar, during the event. This included focus on her clothing, her hand movements, and even the number of times that she blinked during questioning.⁸⁰ But despite this troubling fixation, the press also reliably emphasized how "in control" Sotomayor was during the spectacle.

The theme of restraint was pervasive in the media during the week of the confirmation process, even as the trope of diabetes vanished. The *Washington Post* declared that her "speaking style is deliberate and slow, but she is hardly stiff."⁸¹ The *New York Times* asserted that the Senate panel was balancing a "Tale of Two Sonias." The one who showed up, they argued, "took pains to make herself as boring as possible . . . Not once did she show even a flash of irritation."⁸² She responded to questions "by almost mechanically reciting basic propositions with a controlled and deliberate delivery."⁸³ She was cast as a "thoughtful, cautious jurist who isn't bound by political ideology," offering a "calm, earnest performance" that was "unswoon-worthy."⁸⁴ One journalist took to task Jeffrey Rosen's controversial *New Republic* article by reminding readers about the anonymous sources who lodged accusations against her temperament. That reporter crafted an evocative rejoinder, commenting, "that characterization was called into question by Judge Sotomayor's performance. Despite being questioned aggressively at times, she never got flustered or upset, remaining polite throughout three days of questioning."[85] Rosen himself called her "disciplined and good humored."[86]

Even as diabetes was marginalized as a topic of deliberation during the hearing, previous coverage primed audiences to read the disease as a source of personal control from the start of Sotomayor's journey and was consistently lurking during the confirmation. Glancing through pictures of Sotomayor at the hearing, one can clearly see the customary presence of water glasses that tend to mark bureaucratic events. In several pictures, there are two glasses resting in front of her, which is otherwise unnoticeable in most legislative contexts. One of the glasses, it turns out, was filled with Sprite. Sotomayor kept the soda handy in the event that her sugars plummeted and she needed a quick fix. What is an otherwise invisible disease is given presence, but only slightly, drawing attention to the fact that Sotomayor's condition is always structuring her everyday life and her performance of self. There is no indication that Sotomayor needed to drink the Sprite, again offering a visual testament to the control she has over her body. Diabetes acted as a mechanism for interpreting her disease, and that condition is perpetually in the picture. Diabetes is a paradiscourse, affecting the scene even as it is seemingly absent from the space it occupies. If there are lingering questions about the influence of chronic disease on her persona, we need only turn to the jurist herself, who offered an insightful account of how diabetes management can be understood as acting in concert with abstractions such as wisdom, justice, and decorum.

Diabetes by the Book

In early 2013 Sotomayor released her memoir, *My Beloved World*, an account that concludes just prior to her turbulent Senate confirmation hearings. Unlike the barrage of news stories that used biographical material to introduce her life, Sotomayor begins her narrative by parsing the differences between a memoir and a biography. A memoir, she contends, is more beholden to memory and personal experience and is therefore not an effort to objectively or comprehensibly capture a person's life story. This rhetorically astute crafting allows her to break free from the generic constraints of biography and center her voice after being so tediously scrutinized years earlier by the press and members of Congress. Of course, Sotomayor is one of America's most visible public servants and the book is decidedly political in its scope and aim. It offers a valuable heuristic for reading Sotomayor's nomination, detailing her upbringing and noteworthy academic accomplishments, her amazing career trajectory, and her moderate political disposition. Although the book never reaches the confirmation hearings, the text provides a deft counterpoint to media and congressional narratives that called into question her temperament, affability, and intellect. The memoir both corrects the record and anticipates history's interpretive gaze. Most important for the purposes of this project, Sotomayor's account utilizes anecdotes about diabetes to expound on her life story and cement her reputation as a diligent justice.

My Beloved World is bookended by Sotomayor's experiences with diabetes, wherein each anecdote illustrates her will to live and the vigilant self-care that has been required of her since she was a child. The prologue, to start at one end of the timeline, is an extended meditation about the origins of her diabetes and its role in making her self-sufficient. It opens with a young Sonia waking up to a fight between her parents about which one of them should give her an insulin shot in the days after she is diagnosed. Her father's hands are trembling from the effects of alcoholism and her mother is pleading with him to learn how to administer shots when she is not home. Sotomayor recalls being anxious that she would not be allowed to spend the night at her grandmother's house because of her diabetes and decides then and there, at age eight and in the second grade, to learn how to sterilize needles by boiling them in water and deliver the shots herself. She remembers:

> Watching the water boil would try the patience of any child, but I was as physically restless as I was mentally and had well earned the family nickname Ají—hot pepper—for my eagerness to jump headlong into any mischief impelled by equal parts curiosity and rambunctiousness. But believing that my life now depended on this morning ritual, I would soon figure out how to manage the time efficiently: to get dressed, brush my

teeth, and get ready for school in the intervals while the pot boiled or cooled. I probably learned more self-discipline from living with diabetes than I ever did from the Sisters of Charity.[87]

The contrast between Sotomayor embracing the nickname Ají and the degree of developing self-control alluded to in the anecdote is strikingly similar to the ways diabetes came to act as a containment mechanism in accounts of her experience in the press. It is also reminiscent of the quotation from the confirmation hearing where she contemplated the relationship between emotion and judgment. The various components of her life provided the spiritedness necessary to survive diabetes and retain a sense of independence. It is established from the beginning that Sotomayor finds peace, structure, and ultimately control in ritual and routine. Equally compelling is that Sotomayor embraces her nickname and her "rambunctiousness," showing that restraint and discipline can be expressed in ways that are not beholden to a universal subject typically rendered as white, male, and heterosexual. Protracted discussions of diabetes are rare in the book and occur only at the beginning and ending of the text. Otherwise, diabetes surfaces randomly throughout the memoir, as when Sotomayor would talk about eating sweet mangoes in Puerto Rico, forgetting to eat on the morning of her wedding, and the ways she believed her grandmother was watching over her when she combatted hypoglycemia. But these passages are sporadic and last for only a sentence or two, rarely outlining the ways diabetes shapes daily life. For instance, when Sotomayor recounts walking a mile to school every day, I could not help but think of the numerous times my own sugars had dropped precipitously during a brisk walk. To be sure, Sotomayor likely had scant motivation to detail the mundane realities of diabetes in her memoir. Still, because of this, I believe the places it does surface in her book can offer clues about diabetes's role in shaping the interpretive frame she crafts for reading her legacy.

The second extended anecdote arrives near the text's conclusion and finds Sotomayor having a hypoglycemic attack while celebrating her thirty-seventh birthday at home. Having attended to her guests at the party, she recalls wanting to lie down, only to be approached by a friend who believes she has had too much to drink. Sotomayor remembers grabbing a large piece of birthday cake from her friend's plate and smashing it into her mouth. This visceral scene caught some of her friends off guard because Sotomayor rarely told people about her condition. She writes, "I was averse to any revelations that might have seemed a play for pity. And managing this disease all my life had been the hallmark of self-reliance that had saved me as a child, even if it may have partly cost me a marriage."[88] The rhetorical composition of a diabetic subject is constructed through multiple connections between privacy, constraint, and control. Her determination is marked through the wisdom of a young child, the demise of a relationship, and eventually a seat on the nation's highest court.

Managing diabetes is largely a prudential skill, one that demands practice and situated learning to stay well and stave off complications. After all, medical technologies are only as strong as a person's ability to utilize them properly. Sotomayor grew up in an era when technologies such as glucose monitors and insulin pens and pumps were not readily available. Practicing constraint and discipline were essential because one could not instantly know where blood sugars were resting. She writes, "I cultivated a constant mindfulness of how my body felt. Even now, with much more precise technology at hand, I still find myself mentally checking physical sensations every minute of the day. Along with discipline, that habit of internal awareness was perhaps another accidental gift from my disease. It is linked, I believe, to the ease with which I can recall the emotions attached to memories and to a fine-tuned sensitivity to others' emotional states, which has served me well in the courtroom."[89] This recollection finds kinship with the Obama quotation earlier in this chapter that extols her fortitude and strong will. Disability and perceptiveness are tied together positively—she explicitly calls it a gift—opposing the negative articulation forged between diabetes and her temperament that was present in early press coverage.

The opening and closing anecdotes follow a pattern of pragmatism and self-governing that is ubiquitous in the book. Diabetes literally surrounds her life, cushioning the personal and the political in a sensibility that denotes moderation and deliberation. These rhetorics of balance surface regularly in the text and are a departure from the fiery persona some conservatives tried to assign to her. For example, she writes that she was not enamored of the brash activist tactics she witnessed while at Princeton, noting that political expressions that were too confrontational could "lose potency if used routinely."⁹⁰ She imparts, "Quiet pragmatism, of course, lacks the romance of vocal militancy. But, I felt myself more a mediator than a crusader. My strengths were reasoning, crafting compromises, finding the good and the good faith on both sides of an argument, and using that to build a bridge."⁹¹ Sotomayor is clear that such reflections do not suggest that she cast aside her Latino heritage. At Yale law school, for instance, she found herself with Latinos who "seemed determined to assimilate as quickly and thoroughly as possible, bearing any attendant challenges and psychic costs in private. I could understand the impulse, but it was never a choice I could have made myself."⁹² Sotomayor is equal parts firm in her Puerto Rican background and skeptical of brazen political expression. This moderation is also reflected in her recollections about the formal complaint she filed against an established Washington, DC law firm that suggested she was only admitted to Yale because of affirmative action (as opposed to, for example, graduating summa cum laude from Princeton). Though in the memoir she explicitly chastises the firm for its harassment, the words "racism" and "racist" never appear in the text. She performatively practices the qualities of a Supreme Court justice by avoiding language that might appear indecorous in the context of the political-judicial sphere.

There is also something distinctly queer about Sotomayor, not necessarily her sexuality, but her performance of self and the non-normative ways she has lived her life. She mentions more than once that she lacks a traditionally feminine style and recounts instances when her friends inform her that she acts more like a man than a woman. She vacations on the traditional gay hot spot Fire Island and uses her experiences with diabetes to identify with a cousin who died of AIDS just before his thirtieth birthday. She writes, "I hadn't understood until then that one could be addicted to drugs and yet function normally in the world, holding a job and supporting a family. Nelson [her cousin] wasn't robbing people to get his fix; he wasn't shooting up in stairwells. He managed his addiction like a chronic disease, not unlike my diabetes."⁹³ Sotomayor is acutely aware of the ways supposedly natural, familial bonds are in fact practiced relationalities. The closeness she shares with her mother, for example, is "deeply felt, but we learned it slowly or with effort."⁹⁴ Sotomayor also has deep ambivalence about the institution of marriage, remembering that having a wedding was not as terrible as she believed it would be, but still tells every bride-to-be, "take the money instead."[95] Sad as she was following her divorce, she "was no more sentimental about the formal trappings of marriage than I had been on our wedding day."[96] Although she never had children because of her diabetes, she also believes that the traditional family unit is but one mode of kinship. Families, she rightly scribes, "can be made in other ways, and I marvel at the support and inspiration I've derived from the ones I've built of interlocking circles of friends. In their constant embrace I have never felt alone."[97] If the style of a discourse can reveal the particulars of the subject being produced, this articulation to queerness informs her race, her gender, and her disability in innovative and productive ways. Restraint and self-reliance need not be deterministically normative or blatantly hegemonic. There is in her remarks something creative, fulfilling, and banal all at once.

Diabetes consistently acts as a metaphor for practical wisdom that accentuates the labyrinthine decision-making process of a Supreme Court justice. Sotomayor outlines a number of internal and external factors that she takes into account when administering insulin: "When I'm deciding what I'm going to eat, I calculate the carbohydrate, fat, and protein contents. I ask myself a litany of questions: How much insulin do I need? When is it going to kick in? When was my last shot? Will I walk further than usual or exert myself in a way that might accelerate the absorption rate?"[98] The excessive and chaotic body that is conjoined by disability, gender, and race is articulated to a rational actor who contemplates a series of factors to maintain health.

Still, it should be noted that Sotomayor was not always a study in perfect health. For many years she smoked three and a half packs of cigarettes a day, which is hardly the image of the "good diabetic" found in the media coverage just before her confirmation. She also discussed working at Zaro's Bakery in Co-op City and having a chocolate-covered French cruller every morning for breakfast.[99] I mention these things not to discipline Sotomayor's body, but to note that even as restraint is a defining feature of life with diabetes, there are cracks in the biographical dam. The form of the memoir permits a more compelling and adored subject than the coverage of the judicial hearings, which demanded moderation, thoughtfulness, and a decidedly healthy jurist.

Intersectional Effects and Narrative Remainders

After the White House put forth Sotomayor's name for consideration, the *Washington Post* opened its coverage by remarking, "When President Obama announced his nominee for the Supreme Court last week, he trumpeted her childhood diagnosis of diabetes as one of the challenges she'd overcome. Sonia Sotomayor's success is a testament to how extraordinary life with diabetes can be. Yes, this is a serious disease, without a cure, but it is also very treatable."[100] Diabetes positioned Sotomayor not as a magistrate who was confronting an abbreviated life, but an inspirational figure who transcended adversity through self-discipline. Ultimately these positive qualities inflected a political orientation that conveyed judicial restraint and situational prudence. Diabetes was heralded as a virtue, even if it did not deflect attention away from those aspects of her identity that were attacked relentlessly by members of Congress.

The performative invocations of judiciousness reiterated throughout the vetting process illustrate the rhetorical fungibility of disability. Sotomayor, and by extension her judicial philosophy, were constituted as manageable in order to parlay status and navigate the institutional treachery she confronted. Video archives of the confirmation hearing show Sotomayor taking long pauses, providing thoughtful follow-up information, and rarely flinching in the face of confrontational remarks. Muñoz adduces that this exchange is readily identifiable as a performance by audience members who have lived with the harsh realities of structural and political racism. Like Charles Morris's musings about the fourth persona, Sotomayor's restrained presentation was recognized by those in the know.[101] She was resisting, in Muñoz's words, a *coercive mimesis*, which "understands ethnicity itself as a captivity narrative, one that the minority subject is compelled to perform within" institutions such as the judiciary.[102] She embraced and embodied the shame lobbed at her to generate new conditions of possibility.[103] This performative presentation of self is not one adjudicated solely through race or through gender, but via the complicated interplay of power relations that constituted Sotomayor's persona, which subtly includes her disability.

Sotomayor's character and citizenship were made intelligible through discourses that spotlighted her diabetes, even as the condition appeared to be largely "invisible" throughout the process. Despite this unmarked quality of the disease, Sotomayor and her condition remain decidedly public, being scrutinized and monitored in ways that do not keep pace with cognate cases. Chief Justice Roberts is merely rumored to have epilepsy, without any confirmation or denial that it is real. Everyone knows that Sotomayor has a chronic condition. The high-profile struggles of two other Supreme Court justices, Ruth Bader Ginsburg and Sandra Day O'Connor, fighting cancer is likewise indicative of an ongoing disciplinary pattern that surveils the bodies of women even as men that represent universality, wisdom, and justice, but who might also have health issues, are repeatedly shielded from public appraisals. The effects of discourse materialize incongruently among different bodies. The cultural politics of disease and illness highlight the necessity to further scrutinize disability's byzantine characteristics.

The disciplining of Sotomayor's speech, dress, and persona foretells the ways women, minorities, and those with disabilities are compelled to perform public presentations of self in order to be included in institutional hierarchies. The taming of Sotomayor's appearance mentioned above, for example, was meant to minimize ethnic cues that are coded as contrary to the normative operations of the judicial system. Erin Tarver points out that the White House repeatedly invoked Sotomayor's identity as a "Newyorkrican" to deflect attention from the controversy over her "wise Latina" speech, but also privately instructed her "not to wear her favored hoop earrings or red nail polish to the Senate confirmation hearings."[104] Of course, despite these attempts, Sotomayor was still positioned as uncivil by politicians who argued that she would invite chaos into the legal sphere. The constant gestures toward "restraint" and "balance" become an unfortunate necessity for those who do not occupy a so-called universal subject position. And in this case, the public acclaim that permitted such movement came, in part, from the rhetorical possibilities enabled by her disability.

Finally, in the coverage of Sotomayor's nomination there was an obsessive focus on biography and personal narrative, with little consideration given to systemic failures that marginalize people with diabetes. As a matter of fact, only one news story mentioned insurance when discussing diabetes, which is perhaps the biggest obstacle to maintaining health, especially for those who are socioeconomically disadvantaged.

In this way, we might cautiously approach Sotomayor's success story, because staying well is not generally the product of personal choices or hard work. The fact that Sotomayor grew up in a low-income part of the Bronx in the 1960s might suggest that anyone can overcome the effects of diabetes if only they exhibit enough control. From a public health perspective, this is a risky narrative to impart to low-income populations, especially people of color who struggle with diabetes in disproportionate numbers. According to a report released in 2013, the Bronx had the highest rates of diabetes in New York City, with one in every three residents having the disease. Likewise, in places like East Harlem, where roughly 90 percent of the population is Latino or black, people die from complications related to diabetes at twice the rate of people in the city as a whole.[105] This is not to say that Sotomayor should be chided for her success, only that the media narratives developed around her nomination are not always representative of the experiences of people with diabetes who live in urban enclaves.

Despite these limitations, Sotomayor's story is reparative in many regards and is certainly compelling, if not enviable, because of the ways her disability is recuperated as an aspect of her character not easily compartmentalized from the person she became. Living with diabetes is in fact hard work and Sotomayor continues to set a positive example for many people living with the disease. We must continue telling stories about the discrimination confront by people who occupy complex subject positions to productively transform norms that disparage and discipline some bodies so that others may profit politically, economically, and culturally.

5

Troubled Interventions

"Epidemic" Logic and Institutional Oversight

In 2005, the New York City Department of Health and Mental Hygiene (DOHMH) undertook one of the most far-reaching and ambitious chronic disease intervention programs in the United States. In an effort to combat an alarming surge of diabetes rates among the city's inhabitants, the agency established a patient registry that encouraged New Yorkers to monitor their blood sugar and motivate at-risk residents to visit doctors when glucose levels were precariously elevated. DOHMH required all laboratories serving New York City to report individual A1C scores, which are blood glucose averages for approximately three months, directly to the department so they could start the process of curtailing diabetes's myriad complications. The plan was groundbreaking because for the first time the government would begin tracking individual data about a condition that is neither infectious nor caused by an environmental toxin. Although public health agencies have a long history of intervening in outbreaks like tuberculosis, polio, and yellow fever, this particular resolution was controversial because diabetes is not contagious.[1]

In order to craft comprehensive initiatives that served diverse populations, DOHMH began collecting registry data to "assess variations in testing patterns, health care utilization, and glycemic control" by age, sex, and geographic location.[2] Mapping vectors of excessive glucose results enabled DOHMH to develop broad public health strategies and empower residents to be more conscious of their blood sugars in situ. In this way, the information provided a systemic glance at diabetes and also created opportunities for personal health regimen adjustments. After receiving an A1C score, the department reviewed the data and sent a letter to residents, "informing them of their most recent test result, explaining the risk of complications, and recommending that the patient schedule a return appointment" with their physician.³ The letter, which was written in English and Spanish, provided the recipient with a set of questions to ask doctors and sought to impart a greater sense of agency to New Yorkers when evaluating the status of their health.⁴ The registry also equipped doctors with a quarterly report listing all patients' two most recent A1C scores.⁵

The registry troubled privacy advocates because the collected information would be used to make a direct intervention into the maintenance of a person's health without consent. Proponents of strict medical privacy argued the policy was overly intrusive, even though DOHMH assured registrants that personal information could not be legally disseminated outside the department and would never be used to deny a person employment, healthcare coverage, or driving privileges. Perhaps the most controversial element of the policy stemmed from the fact that people could not opt out of the registry. Patients could stop receiving materials from the city, but all of the previously mentioned information would continue to be sent to the agency. DOHMH defended such measures, contending it could not contemplate workable systemic solutions without a full understanding of diabetes's grip on the city. Privacy advocates retorted that the edict crossed a line, stating the patient-doctor relationship was key to management, not paternalistic intrusion. This stasis point of the debate, pitting the desire of the government to intercede in the treatment of chronic disease against the rights of residents to maintain a reasonable degree of privacy, underscores an important manifestation in public health rhetoric as diabetes becomes more ubiquitous. The competing projections of personal health in the context of communal wellness highlight a schism between liberal conceptions of personal responsibility and civic humanist understandings of public welfare.⁶ Historically, liberalism has been philosophically indebted to a tradition that privileges individual liberties and freedom from state regulation. Civic humanism, conversely, emphasizes civic virtue, public action, and the common good. Elements of each can be traced in contemporary American culture and their components are best understood as motivating political impulses, not wholly discreet worldviews. I appropriate and scrutinize aspects of these broad heuristics to unpack arguments about New York City's controversial measure and yet another orientation for contemplating diabetes management: community action.

At the heart of this conversation is the changing nature of healthcare strategies in America and the ever-increasing ability to manage once-deadly diseases. Former DOHMH Commissioner Dr. Thomas Frieden (who was later appointed head of the Center for Disease Control by President Obama) argued that public health officials had been "asleep at the switch," noting that "local health departments generally do a good job of monitoring and controlling conditions that killed people in the United States 100 years ago. Yet noncommunicable diseases, which accounted for less than 20 percent of US deaths in 1900, now account for about 80 percent of deaths. Our local public health infrastructure has not kept pace with this transition."[7] The extension of the human life span necessitates a continual rethinking of the mission of public health departments and the ways bureaucracies imagine populations to justify intervention strategies. The budding preponderance of noncommunicable diseases and the interdependent ethics of care they demand as a result are of great consequence for policy makers seeking a balance between state influence and personal autonomy.

In this chapter I explore the implications stemming from the tension between individual agency and institutional regard, looking at a dual emphasis on public intervention and personal privacy in noncommunicable diseases like diabetes. DOHMH positions diabetes in a manner that mirrors infectious disease, revealing the extent to which surveillance might act as a strategy for "containment" in popular scientific vernacular. The department stresses the concept of the "epidemic," giving the presumed excesses of diabetes new urgency and offering an alternative to the rhetorical sedimentation that typically characterizes the condition. Unlike the previous chapter, which accentuated perseverance and personal transcendence, the epidemic metaphor is collective in its epistemological impulse, offering the rhetorical resources to engage conceptions of disease in ways that singular notions of sovereignty occlude. The image of diabetes as an "epidemic" implies large-scale quantities of people struggling with disease, but without the baggage of being labeled a "contagion." This strategic discourse has the productive effect of mobilizing the resources to contest diabetes rates. However, if misdirected it could also reinscribe notions of individual fortitude over aggressive structural change. This is especially worrisome because DOHMH's model, which is dependent on knowledge *after* diagnosis, continues to pose challenges for implementing preventative measures at the local level. The department's early emphasis on monitoring and controlling disease rarely addressed the most essential cultural changes required for eradicating diabetes. Nonetheless, I contend in this chapter that the registry is an important step in recognizing diabetes as a social ill that can be cooperatively defeated.

Narrating the early history of clinical health, Michel Foucault noted that the institution emerged from a "medicine of epidemics," remarking that whether contagious or not an epidemic has an "historical individuality, hence the need to employ a complex method of observation when dealing with it."[8] The contention that epidemics are intimately political and can be figuratively appropriated to discipline and control people has been widely documented, and scholars ranging from Susan Sontag to Pricilla Wald have provided ample reason to be suspicious of the frame.[9] Taking a page from Foucault's later writings on discourse, however, this chapter analyzes the civic potential of the metaphor of "epidemic," recognizing that trajectories of discourse are not always easily delimited. In the specific instance of the debate over the New York City registry, the metaphor may help shift conceptions of diabetes from being a privately managed disease to a condition that is collectively managed. While keeping concerns about state overreach present, I argue the metaphor of "epidemic" might enable societal transformation, allowing officials to corral resources to curtail diabetes rates. Despite the recalcitrance toward "epidemic" as a trope, it remains more empowering than invocations of privacy, which are entirely impotent, purporting to support actions that save people with diabetes, but which secure a model that renders the disease a product of individual maintenance and discipline, not social reform. Those forwarding privacy claims are not mindful of how their assertions resituate diabetes as an individualized disease, fortifying the quandary diabetes advocates seek to subsume.

These two factions, however, do not necessarily represent wholly disparate positions. While "epidemics" and "medical privacy" appear to reproduce an old divide between public and private, they share a focus on modalities of treatment in the forms of prevalence and personal data that bring this debate to life in problematic ways. Those residents most marginalized by the condition, including those who have no health care, can be inadvertently erased in prevalence reports. New York City officials have a more productive civic strategy, but a rhetorical approach that invigorates isolationist management practices must be avoided for the endeavor to be revelatory.[10] Of course, one undertaking cannot circumvent deeply ingrained cultural habits and systemic failures, such as our inability to launch single-payer health care in the United States. New York City's registry is but one sign, albeit a promising one, that diabetes can be socially addressed and cooperatively constrained.

Start Spreading the News

The history of public health surveillance in America is marked by a tension between the desire to keep communities healthy and simultaneously respect the privacy of residents whenever possible. Although it is easy to conceptualize this dichotomy in traditional political terms, accentuating the conservative tendency to value libertarian individualism versus progressive notions of government intercession, public health policy is vastly more complicated, especially when we consider the evolution of privacy, the stigma attached to particular diseases, and the changing nature of what constitutes a public danger. There has long existed a dialogical antagonism in surveillance between the promise of disease control and the prospect of institutional intrusion.[11] This friction is especially pronounced with regard to disease registries because associating particular individuals or groups to conditions such as tuberculosis or HIV can incite or increase feelings of social impurity. So far, this book has discussed the diffuse ways that diabetes is publicly characterized as easily managed, inevitably fatal, or individually transcended. In the case of New York City's intervention project we find a return to ruinous rhetoric, much like that of the JDRF, but one underscored by a reparative frame that suggests sweeping reforms can improve collective health.[12]

The uptake of cataclysmic rhetoric is not surprising when we consider just how lethal diabetes is in New York City, where almost 90 percent of adults diagnosed with the disease do not know their A1C scores.[13] Between 1990 and 2003, the death rate from diabetes in the five boroughs rose by more than 70 percent.[14] Two public health experts reflected on the startling nature of the evidence at the time the municipality moved to put its registry into place:

In New York City alone, an estimated 530,000 people have diagnosed and 265,000 have undiagnosed diabetes. Approximately 1800 deaths and 1700 amputations as well as other complications add up to an $8.3 billion cost in New York City. Among the elderly and some minorities, the prevalence is between 12% and 20%. It is predicted that 30% to 50% of today's children may develop diabetes.[15]

This information is further confounded by the fact that New Yorkers with diabetes are hospitalized at a rate nearly 80 percent higher than the national average. Along with the emotional, physical, and mental impact the disease has had on residents in the city, it has also proven to be expensive. The price of diabetic hospitalizations doubled to $481 million in 2003, just two years before the registry was launched, up from $242 million thirteen years earlier.[16] Today those figures remain staggeringly high. Despite rising costs, people with diabetes are spending less time in hospitals for treatment and care.[17]

Studies have also found that, for a variety of reasons, a number of subpopulations and minorities in New York are especially hard hit by diabetes. African Americans, Puerto Ricans, and Russian-speaking immigrants all have high rates of diabetes. Asian New Yorkers are more likely than any other ethnicity to have pre-diabetes.[18] The pilot program for the New York City registry began in the South Bronx, where 48,000 adults have been diagnosed and a quarter of those are classified in the danger zone of having "poorly controlled diabetes."[19] DOHMH defines a hazardous A1C score as anything above 9 percent, which is an average glucose reading of 212. These statistics are compounded by the poverty rate in New York City, which stands at over 20 percent, much higher than the national rate of just under 13 percent.[20] Since the genesis of the registry, DOHMH officials have launched studies to assess how care for underserved populations can be more effectively administered in order to save lives.[21]

Registries create a link between the surveillance of a disease and patient care. In the state of New York there are registries for cancer, Alzheimer's, congenital malformations, communicable diseases, lead poisoning, and immunizations.[22] However, in the case of the city's diabetes initiative, observers noted that "no health department has ever sought to exercise such thorough influence over care that it does not directly provide."[23] DOHMH leaders contended that these inventories serve an important function because they offer "a mechanism by which providers can identify individuals in greatest need of follow-up or referral and also monitor disease indicators in their patient population over time."[24] There is evidence that registries can have a positive impact on patient health, but even the most well-known surveillance campaigns raise questions about the motivations of patients, the treatments received, and the privileged position of benefactors.[25]

The diabetes registry is intended to spark awareness about the everyday ramifications of the disease and move conversations that are shaded by stigma into the light. Public health officials are faced with the challenge of crafting programs that empower residents, but without the guilt and remorse that tends to accompany diabetes, especially for those living with type 2. A sense of urgency must also be ignited to combat the steady march of the disease for those with persistently high numbers and the ensuing feelings of being overpowered. When executed properly, registries can provide elastic rubrics for wellness that refrain from overly intrusive judgments about personal habits, routines, or cultural traditions. There is no denying that the model being advocated by DOHMH would be best fulfilled by activated patients who can apply broad principles to specific situations. But unanimous compliance is unlikely and surveillance techniques will never capture the nuances of day-to-day life for each resident. As a result, there will always be gaps between how state actors imagine the ideal actions of people with diabetes and actual lived practices. The map simply does not always reflect the territory. Like other illness experiences, people with diabetes will evaluate their struggles in *particularistic* terms, while institutional medicine will assess it in *universal* terms.[26] Despite these tensions, registries might envision collectives in a more innovative fashion than is typically done by those invested in care regimens. It is in this vein that the metaphor of "epidemic" becomes fruitfully pragmatic.

Constituting the "Epidemic"

The role of language in bringing to life medical abstractions is an essential feature of public health rhetorics. Far from being merely descriptive, language and tropes such as metaphors give form to ephemeral aspects of culture, performing what some have called a "constitutive" function in materializing accepted "truths." Language offers presence to unseen illnesses and allows for the communal contemplation of otherwise abstract ideas. The shared meanings that physicians, patients, and those invested in management routines ascribe to wellness and illness can initiate possibilities for understanding affective phenomena and orient attitudes for plotting public health strategies. Commenting on the relationship between language and the materialization of collective realities, Judy Segal has noted, "the outcomes of health-policy debate are constrained in part by the biomedical terms and metaphors in which the debate takes place."[27] Giving attention to the contingent terminologies that structure medicine and public health emphasizes their composition as a constellation of "norms and values operating discursively" alongside the biological workings of the endocrine system.[28] Of course, such framing does not exist in a vacuum. The scope of public health rhetoric is dependent on the contexts in which it emerges, the privileging of particular terms at opportune moments, and the attitudes that such communication inspires.[29]

Public health discourses facilitate this constitutive function, engendering communal identities in the midst of crises. Metaphors and narratives influence how those practicing medicine and "lay" publics understand the consequences of disease, how they perceive threats to the community, and how they conceive solutions.[30] As has been noted elsewhere in this book, metaphors that naturalize the idea of "combatting" or "fighting" diseases such as cancer are not merely descriptive, but can have serious consequences on how patients process illness and internalize feelings of isolation and shame should treatments fail. As noted earlier in this text, however, those same metaphors can be strategically adopted in a different context and put to good use, as was the case with the JDRF. The relational logic of terms, Priscilla Wald has observed, "runs much deeper than state mechanisms and inflects the conception of community articulated in the narratives."[31] Rhetorics such as outbreak narratives "actually make the act of imagining the community a central (rather than obscured) feature of its preservation." Nancy Tomes contends that the norms born of such languages are negotiated in the relationship among medical and public health institutions and those contending with illness in everyday life. In short, meanings are intellectually dynamic, not distortions of pure scientific knowledge.

Tomes asserts, "scientific precepts become a part of the working hypothesis of everyday life" because "no disease is ever observed in a totally unbiased way; there is always a scrim of culture affecting our perceptions of and attempts to treat illness."[32] The frames adopted to process public health crises directly correspond to how we respond to such emergencies.

Public health agencies frequently adapt their rhetorical strategies to justify controversial measures.[33] Even when citizens support the actions of a department or when agencies are afforded legal backing, officials employ language to already accepted cultural frames to promote campaigns that may be contentious. It comes as little surprise, then, that DOHMH has appropriated the conceptual heuristic of "epidemic" to assert the import of the registry and convey the high stakes of successfully implementing the operation. Citizens have been primed to see the continued relationship between diabetes, obesity, and personal responsibility, and it is this "crisis" that has given rise to the necessity of government intervention.[34] Indeed, so common is the signifying power of this discourse that Lisa Keränen has demonstrated that we are now living with an "epidemic of epidemics."[35] The frame of "epidemic" is especially pragmatic in two senses: First, it offers urgency to seemingly mundane conditions that might actually be hazardous to public health. Second, although an epidemic model is popularly associated with communicable diseases, it also has the capacity to spotlight systemic ills and thereby commence conversations about bureaucratic solutions.

The word "epidemic" is scattered throughout the literature engaging the registry. It appeared on the DOHMH website when the venture was initiated, was used in materials residents could download from the agency, and is commonly invoked by city spokespeople. For example, in a publication defending the plan, DOHMH officials noted, "In December 2005, *in characterizing diabetes as an epidemic*, the New York City Board of Health mandated the laboratory reporting of hemoglobin A1C laboratory test results."[36] The word "epidemic" appears at strategic moments in the DOHMH article, but tellingly, twice in the abstracts (once in the context abstract, once in the conclusions abstract) and twice again in final paragraph. For readers skimming the report, the placement of the word is easily identified and drives home the point that diabetes is at critical levels and necessitates immediate action.

The incorporation of the term "epidemic" constitutes the consequences of diabetes's tumultuous character, delimiting both a confounding crisis and possibilities for public responses. Etymologically, the word "epidemic" means "on the people" and carries with it the notion of a condition necessitating relief.[37] One public heath advocate contended that by labeling diabetes as an epidemic, doctors could "develop public health strategies to prevent or reverse obesity and physical inactivity with the goal of decreasing the development of diabetes and its complications," adding that, "without surveillance, it is going to be very hard to tackle the problem."[38] Epidemics, after all, "require bold public health action."[39] The framing of diabetes as an epidemic also had the effect of making it populist in nature: Disease is not discriminatory through this lens. As Gordon Mitchell and Kathleen McTigue point out, invoking the term epidemic encourages people to view such issues "as a matter of common concern, not a condition afflicting a few isolated individuals."[40] Or, as Wald puts it, epidemics "dramatize the need for regulation."[41] Epidemics require immediate attention from the state so the disease can be monitored and eventually eradicated.

Dr. Shadi Chamany, the director of the New York City Diabetes Prevention Program, has insisted that the framing of diabetes as an epidemic was not strategic, but simply a term utilized by public health advocates. In an interview she explained to me:

> I think the term "epidemic," some people are very uncomfortable with that word. But it is epidemic. I think in practicing good public health, we are describing a problem that is epidemic. It's growing. It's affecting more and more of the population. There's no other motive for using that term other than just to describe it. We could say in "characterizing the problems of diabetes increasing rapidly," but I think it's very descriptive. It's a term we use in public health. I do think people have associations with it sometimes that . . . can be kind of scary. You know, when you hear "epidemic" you can think of an outbreak [or] something like that. But it doesn't always have to apply to something that's, you know, right there and it's an infectious disease outbreak. There wasn't any particular reason for us using that word other than it's a term we use in public health.

Here, "epidemic" is characterized in a manner described by Cindy Patton as "apparently simple." It is "more cases of a disease than expected."[42] Regardless of the seemingly conscious opening line of the report that explicitly references the overt characterizing of diabetes as an epidemic, the frame is taken to be a natural extension of public health vernacular. Nonetheless, instinctively adopting this designation is equally striking. The appropriation designates an acceptable frame that is accessible, ubiquitous, and powerful.[43] Epidemic here toggles between being an expression of art for public health practitioners and a term that residents can process with ease.

The very suggestion of epidemic connotes urgency, which public health officials frequently see as lacking in patient attitudes about diabetes. The gradual onset of complications from diabetes often causes those living with the disease to distance themselves from a language that emphasizes imminent harm because the effects of rising sugar levels colonize the body slowly. Like many chronic diseases, there is a lack of exigency for receiving care. The language of epidemics offers health operatives a critical frame for reorienting the disease as a *crisis*. If we understand a crisis as a breakdown in meaning, then inciting projections of peril allows for the resignification of chronic disease as a concern to be addressed promptly. As DOHMH pointed out in its initial report, "Resistance to New York City's public health approach to diabetes control may result at least in part from the continued attribution of the current epidemic to individual genetic susceptibility and personal lifestyle choices, neither of which invokes a sense of urgency or validates public health response."[44] Others in the debate echoed this sentiment, asserting, "patients lack a sense of urgency for the treatment of their chronic disease and also sense a lack of efficacy of many interventions."[45] This need not mean that people with diabetes are lazy (though such insinuations are frequent), only that the malaise of daily routines quickly dissipates the imminence of potential consequences.

The need for institutional actors to instigate a sense of urgency is regarded as especially critical in relation to obesity, which is always suggested in diabetes discourse, even when it is not publicly stated or contextually appropriate. The articulation of obesity with the trope of "epidemic" is persistent in American culture, constructing a frame that allows for diabetes to be incorporated into the parameters of public health logics. This is certainly true in the medical literature, where articles such as "The Continuing Epidemics of Obesity and Diabetes in the United States" often circulate.[46] This metaphor is equally prevalent in broader public spheres. A good example is provided in a *Newsweek* editorial penned by First Lady Michelle Obama in March 2010. She writes:

> For years, we've known about the *epidemic* of childhood obesity in America. We've heard the statistics—how one-third of all kids in this country are either overweight or obese. We've seen the effects on how our kids feel, and how they feel about themselves. And we know the risks to their health and to our economy—the billions of dollars we spend each year treating obesity-related conditions like heart disease, *diabetes*, and cancer.[47]

Again, we should not forget that epidemics are often imagined as populist in nature, with the potential to harm anyone, hence the First Lady's emphasis on the contraction "we've" three times in three sentences. Obesity here is collectively related to a number of conditions where the effects are clearly damaging. Obama's words also hint at the potential of employing the word epidemic counterintuitively, wherein institutional resources might be marshaled and productive interventions realized. Despite the identification of ills that may stem from obesity, the solutions that are eventually offered in the editorial do not achieve similar effect in their reconciliation of the predicament. The gradualism of the problem, its cause, and solutions simply do not fit popular understandings of "epidemics." Sander Gilman has commented that the First Lady's conceptualization of obesity and diabetes as a consequence of "laziness" illustrates how easily even well-intentioned discourse slips back into a language that emphasizes individual fortitude and personal responsibility.[48] Especially since we know not all fat bodies will develop diabetes, including the majority of those classified as obese, we would be wise to push on the limits of this metaphor and its public circulation.

Along with a heightened sense of urgency, the frame of "epidemic" has a second important function: It draws attention to communal harms that transcend personal struggles. In this manner, it might be useful to follow diabetes in vectors, to trace it with maps and charts in ways that mimic more traditional understandings of epidemics. Certainly, such vectors can determine the prevalence of disease and lay a path for policy reforms. On a more pessimistic note, diabetes is attended to in the DOHMH plan in a largely reactionary fashion, being addressed only after diagnosis. When public officials argue that surveillance is essential for "identifying clusters, mapping the spread of disease, understanding patterns of contagion, and detecting lapses in hospital infection control," the limitations of the registry must be pondered.[49] Diabetes does not map well on to any of these.

While bold intervention is no doubt compelling in an age when chronic diseases are killing the vast majority of citizens, an important distinction needs to be made between the mapping of infectious and non-infectious conditions. Outbreaks of infectious diseases can generally be contained in a relatively short period of time after their trajectory is determined. Diabetes has no such travel plans. Maps produced by the city are always signifying something else, exacerbating the degree to which diabetes is *not* mobile. These vectors, unlike their communicable counterparts, are relatively stable and predictable. Despite their immobility, history tells us that residents are still likely to be shunned as living without personal restraint and excessively transcending the medical order, especially by moralizers who subscribe to unreflective scripts of individual responsibility. If infectious disease tells us something about how a disease travels, then assuredly these new maps tell us something about how diabetes is remarkably stationary.

This geographic focus suggests that diabetes is always contained, but not by the confinement of bodies in quarantine. These are people isolated by poverty and those who lack medical care. These vectors of disease evidence the structural ordering of food choices (or lack thereof), the ability of people to access medical attention, and the capacity to digest the emotional, physical, and cultural aspects of living with diabetes. As two public health officials put it:

> Simply knowing A1C levels is clearly not sufficient. It is not enough for the patient to "know their numbers" if they do not have the knowledge, resources, or skills to do anything about it. It is not enough for the provider to know the numbers if insufficient resources are allocated to optimize disease management. Resources for diabetes management include safe areas for walking and other physical activity and afford-

able nutritional options, as well as affordable medications and glucose monitoring devices. Even these are insufficient if society promotes excess food consumption, including sugary drinks, and if healthy affordable food choices of fruits and vegetables are unavailable. In a city with a large immigrant population, food security is an important issue; as people migrate from areas of food scarcity to areas of abundance, the tendency is to overeat, which results in increased rates of obesity and diabetes. Alternatives for healthy eating might also enlist the support of local farms to promote use of fresh, tasty food.[50]

The data are never pointing simply to bodies so much as they are to systemic concerns that must be addressed by government programs, collective action, medical resolve, and a healthcare system that privileges people and not profits. As Patton notes, epidemiology must "constantly construct and correlate populations and subpopulations in order to make epidemics visible—hence its reliance on the descriptive and predictive technologies of surveillance and sentinel studies."[51] In the case of diabetes, these bodies are signs of man-made vexations including available food choices, medical accessibility, and the luxury to make healthy lifestyle decisions such as exercising.

The lack of collective urgency underwriting diabetes and its stationary nature hints at the ways chronic disease temporally molds public health agendas. Just as blood sugars rise incrementally, systems and habits both solidify gradually. Changing life for people with diabetes is difficult without reforms in other areas of public culture, including early detection plans that will remain out of reach for many as long as economically marginalized populations are denied regular contact with a physician. People often live for a decade without knowing blood sugar levels are slowly killing them. Surveillance cannot be contained to individual bodies, but must look to arenas of life that enable diabetes and its ramifications to manifest undetected and unchecked. Even with this knowledge, there is reason to be hesitant about the relationship between bodies, geography, and the epidemic frame. The very presence of high A1C scores collected by DOHMH suggests that people are receiving care. Prevalence is dependent on medical detection and those areas most in need of help may long be underrepresented. As Chamany reflected:

> [W]here are the people who have very high A1Cs? We imagine they'll probably be in the same places where we have very high prevalence. But we don't know that. We should look at it. It may be more scattered across the city. You know, maybe the difficulty in getting control isn't necessarily where the highest prevalence is. We don't know that. We can take a look at patterns of where people are getting their tests, how often people are going to the same doctor versus not.

In short, prevalence is significant to mapping the epidemic, but it is also reliant on residents being diagnosed with diabetes—perhaps years too late. Identifying diabetes can still be a positive outcome for initiating the long process of collectively diminishing the condition, but the poorest of areas might rest beyond the reach of the registry to start.

Despite the limits of DOHMH's rhetoric, its emphasis on publics in the debate over the registry situates it as a decidedly forward-looking enterprise. Appeals to privacy rarely address the public good, perpetually imagining a diabetic body that is sovereign and detached from cultural contexts. These overtures to privacy also contend that any form of health care performed outside the physician's office, including those advocated by agencies such as DOHMH, is generally detrimental. In the next section, I explore arguments from privacy advocates to delimit their understanding of diabetes, interventions, and public life.

Privacy and the Frame of Civil Rights

The histories of medicine and public health are littered with examples that illustrate the deleterious invasion of a person's privacy in the name of the greater good. A cursory glance at AIDS's devastating history, for example, highlights the dual struggle to ensure people receive care but also that their personal information is protected from intrusion. Too often patients have been made to fight for the right to be left alone, against the state and healthcare providers, as they attempt to stay well. This "democratic privacy" is a productive exercise in motivating activated citizens, but usually comes only after much struggle and often much heartache.[52] To be clear, I believe privacy appeals are persuasive and should be taken seriously to protect the rights of residents. However, claims to privacy must be engaged to ensure that such arguments do not strip already disadvantaged populations of access to medicine, care, and community. Declarations rooted in maximizing privacy rights can easily slip into abstracted notions of personhood and problematically universalize the ability of local inhabitants to stay well.

As mentioned at the start of this chapter, DOHMH's plan was unusually contentious because it was compulsory and disallowed residents to opt out of the program. The controversy surrounding informed consent made it particularly surprising, then, that none of the major organizations dedicated to privacy participated in the debates leading up to the implementation of the registry.[53] As Amy Fairchild, Ronald Bayer, and James Colgrove note, the city "did not initially consult the county, state, and national medical associations. Given the sensitivity of surveillance surrounding HIV case reporting, it is likewise striking that privacy advocates were not included in early discussions" prior to the debates.[54] The department did, however, hold public hearings about the plan, allowing for the parameters of the program to be amended. Still, such oversights likely furthered some suspicions of the registry, making people skeptical of its otherwise laudable goals. Privacy becomes a blanket defense to what is perceived as poor planning, even when health officials appear to be proceeding with admirable intentions.

People living with diabetes often prize privacy because of the stigma and blame attached to the disease. It is worth repeating that those with diabetes are constantly reminded that they need to carefully manage their blood sugar to stay well. If they do not, they alone are seen as responsible for their demise. This pervasive misperception about the ways diabetes functions, along with poor understandings of medicines such as insulin, make individuals with diabetes easy targets for public scapegoating. The American Diabetes Association (ADA) receives approximately 200 calls each month about discrimination in schools, the workplace, and correctional institutions.[55] It is for this reason the ADA's executive committee was reluctant to endorse the city's initial policy, supporting surveillance only if the patient offered affirmative consent each time bloodwork was completed.[56]

A number of critics weighed in on the precedent being set by the registry. For some, the new undertaking was reproducing the egregious harms that the ADA fights so hard to prevent. Janlori Goldman, a faculty member at the Center for the History and Ethics of Public Health and Department of Sociomedical Sciences at Columbia, wrote, these "initiatives do not balance heightened surveillance and intervention with the provision of meaningful safeguards or resources for prevention and treatment."[57] Harold Krent, a dean at Chicago-Kent school of law, proclaimed, "the A1C registry will be used to supervise the non-criminal behavior of private citizens, namely, how well diabetics are managing their own blood sugar levels."[58] Margaret Hoppin took up the registry to coin the phrase "emergent public health surveillance" and express concern about a security state run amok, one that would employ extra-legal data-mining techniques to target politically vulnerable communities.[59] Finally, Wendy Mariner of Boston University's schools of Public Health and Law contended that the city "fails to satisfy basic legal principles governing patient autonomy and privacy."[60] These sentiments were reflected by some citizens during the public hearings, who asked, "Are you going to demand what I can and can't eat?"[61]

The reservations raised by privacy advocates are compelling and merit serious reflection. It is not my intention here to call into question the motives of these scholars and advocates. I believe each of them has genuine concerns about patient privacy. Rather, I hope to scrutinize the degree of agency they contend to be offering people with diabetes, as their visions often work to privatize disease, deflecting attention away from systemic issues and back on to the individual body. Unlike the public character of the ailment put forth by the city, these declarations reproduce the notion that diabetes merely necessitates personal management. To expand on this point, I turn to critiques made by Goldman, Hoppin, Krent, and Mariner, focusing on the frame of privacy, their concerns about government overreach, and the consequential individuation of disease. I give attention to each of these figures in part because their writings are thoughtful appraisals of the registry, but also because their publications have steadily built from one another to establish a case against New York City's project. As the following pages explain, I do not disagree with every characterization they make, though I certainly allow more license to DOHMH's mandate.

First, these scholars worried that DOHMH was overreaching in its mission and that patients would have their personal data manipulated (if not outright stolen) by agencies and their workers. Krent and colleagues, for example, were troubled by the potential use of the registry for future research without the consent of those enrolled in the program.[62] They alleged that the registry gives public health officials unlimited access to people's medical histories without prior consent. They cited a number of concerns, including disclosure in relation to new disability policies, the prospect of hackers, and employees who would sell information for a profit.[63] Krent and affiliates went as far as to argue that a registry notification would "create a new affirmative duty in the patient" to disclose a diabetes diagnosis or their poor management of the disease when applying for services or a job.[64] Hoppin likewise voiced apprehension about the potential to further gather personal data, alleging that the city was opening the floodgates for the government to commandeer information from unsuspecting residents. The data from continuous glucose monitors (CGMs), for example, "could be made available to public health agencies with minimal additional cost and few logistical implications."[65] Neither DOHMH nor any other agency has expressed such intent, but there remained concerns that the municipality could stretch it surveillance techniques as broadly as they saw fit without the worry of strict legal scrutiny. The registry, in this work, constitutes a new legal subjectivity whose publicness is inherently risky.[66]

Echoes of liberalism permeate this discourse, with tropes of freedom and individual responsibility actualizing contractual legal metaphors.[67] These appeals are not surprising in the context of law journals, but they have the effect of circumscribing complex cultural issues into narrowed constructions of "the state" (which is generally positioned as menacing) and the "individual" (typically seen as vulnerable). Hoppin suggested that management is left to the latter and reducible to personal decisions "about behavior and lifestyle—what to eat, how much stress to accept in jobs or personal life, how much exercise, and what portion of limited time and energy to devote to health management."[68] The emphasis on how much stress "to accept" points to the ways individuals are imagined as empowered free of contextual circumstances such as employment insecurity or a stifled job market. She goes on to claim that the registry targets "lifestyle" conditions, in part because she is focused on privacy considerations stemming from the Fourth and Fourteenth amendments to the US Constitution. Importantly, the registry does not focus on specific choices—it focuses on A1C scores, which are broad signposts for glucose levels, not daily activity trackers.

Mariner likewise expressed skepticism of the plan, noting that the city had not met the basic requirements of legality to ensure that patient data has been protected. She argued:

> [W]hat begins as a benevolent effort to encourage better medical care may mutate into requiring compliance with a medical regimen as a condition for Medicaid eligibility, private health insurance, public or private employment, or even the general duty to stay healthy. A disproportionate number of diabetics in New York City are Medicaid beneficiaries or disadvantaged minorities and the City would benefit financially from any reduction in the cost of their care.[69]

The undercurrent of liberalism, wherein the "duty" to stay well is a "mutation" from a more organic state, is typical of a language strategy that portrays these interventions as inherently contractual and not actually benevolent. As I have noted, people with diabetes repeatedly internalize a moral obligation to be healthy, even when they do not have access to lifesaving technologies. This is especially true for residents with scant resources and who are alienated by a rhetoric that emphasizes "freedom" from health care. So, while it may be true that the city would benefit from a decrease in costs, there is no evidence that officials wished to further marginalize people in need. A far greater concern might be the reintroduction of a language of management that leaves people isolated. The claims about medical qualifications and pre-existing conditions are negated by the Affordable Care Act as of this writing, but deserve ongoing attention should Donald Trump's administration decide to repeal the law.[70] Such an action would no doubt be devastating to millions of people. For those who already have insurance the claim is completely negligible because, as Krent notes, "an insurer would likely have access to A1C test results regardless of whether that information is tracked in the registry. Health insurance companies have broad rights to inspect medical information in order to evaluate medical claims."[71] Each of the quandaries outlined above already exists in some form, and staying the course with current policies would not effectively alter the trajectory of treatment.[72]

Critics maintained concern that the registry unnecessarily lengthened the reach of the government in an era when the full effects of the Patriot Act are still being weighed. Especially since diabetes is not contagious, expanding the powers of the state seemed to them wrongheaded. Looking to the tuberculosis registry created by New York City officials in the nineteenth century, Hoppin concurred that such ventures were successful, but that the analogy to present-day noncommunicable diseases should be treated with suspicion. She writes, "The innovations—and the problems—at the heart of emergent programs are that they target individuals who pose no health risk to others, and they employ technology that enables surveillance that is virtually unlimited in scope."[73] Mariner claims that the law has always been an effective tool to implement public health policy, but that the measure is nonetheless invasive.[74] She suggests that laws governing sewage, food, drugs, and vaccinations have a public character not shared by diabetes: "Yet, where the state overrides an individual's right to information privacy, it requires specific justification beyond general appeals to improve health."[75] The constitutive feature of this rhetoric, wherein diabetes is subsumed to the legal category of "information privacy" and simultaneously without "public" character, illustrates a complete vanishing of the condition in this rhetoric.

Both Mariner and Hoppin found the expanded concepts of "epidemics" and "disease surveillance" particularly troublesome. The former notes that the metaphors "encourage the notion that health departments are entitled to personally identifiable health information about everyone in the state."[76] Epidemics, she laments, are now defined as "any increase in the number of people with a particular disease or condition that is higher than would be expected based on past experience. Thus, we read news reports of an epidemic of obesity or breast cancer."[77] Speaking directly to the need for a more nuanced lexicon, she contended that the "absence of language explaining why one disease or condition differs from any other makes it difficult to determine the limits of any principle being applied."[78] Mariner raises an important point when she observes, "We've begun to talk about chronic diseases in the same way we talk about contagious diseases, and so it follows that we would start to take the same kind of public health measures."[79] Following this line of thought, Hoppin writes that those who employ the word "epidemic" are too quick to see commonalities among diabetes and infectious disease and that further scrutiny should be given to the analogy. Like those in the second chapter who insist no logical associations exist among HIV and diabetes, Hoppin encourages readers to jettison the comparison. Echoing Chamany's words during our interview, Hoppin vies, "But diabetes is like an infectious disease only in the sense that it is widespread and increasingly prevalent. Unlike infectious disease, it cannot be 'stopped' by government intervention in the lives of people who have it."[80] Of course, without the administration of such endeavors, officials are left with little data to produce strategies for addressing the preponderance of diabetes rates in the city. What is overlooked here is that "epidemic" provides wide cultural and legal latitude to agencies eager to provide assistance. While the frame of "epidemic" can be employed in draconian fashion, it can also be utilized to resituate diabetes rates as a predicament necessitating urgent action and resources. Not all government intervention need be biopolitical in only its negative sense.

To resist the positioning of diabetes as a publicly motivated concern, a recurrent argument surfaces that resituates the site of privacy in the physician's office, between the doctor and patient. This theme has a long history in public health debates. At the end of the nineteenth century through the start of the twentieth century, language emphasizing the idea of "privacy" was primarily employed by physicians. When New York began collecting information on tuberculosis in 1897, "physicians resisted on the basis that patient privacy might be violated."[81] Well over a century later, such sentiments lingered when the diabetes registry was proposed. For instance, the Association of American Physicians and Surgeons, an "organization opposed to the 'evil' of government based or 'socialized' medicine, objected to lab-based A1C reporting as a 'blatant invasion of patient privacy that will cause many patients to avoid testing and treatment."[82] This hyperbolic claim, which creates an unfounded slippery slope, assumes that current individual management practices—including those for people without health care—are sufficient for treating diabetes. In most cases, they are not.

Those writing in opposition to DOHMH frequently foreground structural solutions to diabetes, but generally retreat into claims about privacy violations as their arguments progress. The public character of diabetes is noted but never sufficiently addressed in ways that would aid residents grappling with the disease. For example, beginning with an argument about the systematic nature of diabetes, Goldman slowly spirals into an individualized notion of disease. Institutional alterations are hinted at, but no solutions for alleviating the municipality's dilemmas are given. Goldman writes:

> the underlying social, environmental, and economic factors that contribute to disease must be confronted, and the doctor–patient relationship must be reinforced with resources that enhance treatment, communication, and trust. In the zeal to ameliorate pressing health problems, public health measures may alienate the very communities and health professionals they aim to serve and reduce a willingness to seek or to provide health care services.[83]

The system is mentioned but never attended to in a way that might actually assuage the distress experienced by people with diabetes. Because Goldman situates the disease in the private sphere, little can be done to elucidate and modify its public character. She continues, "although the DOHMH sees a duty to intervene for a population that is economically and medically vulnerable, this same population—as the target of the pilot intervention—is especially concerned about the risk of stigma, discrimination, and a 'blame-the-victim' approach to the disease."[84] However, in rendering diabetes private, Goldman concurrently marginalizes the shame and stigma experienced by people who live with the disease. That is, shame and stigma are not alleviated, but merely moved out of sight. Goldman sees every player in the game as a loser in this formulation: physicians, patients, and even public health officials. Still, her claims that the program will "further erode trust and confidence in public health officials" seem baseless without presenting empirical evidence that residents will recoil at a registry designed to provide aid.[85]

DOHMH pushed back on the idea that the city was attempting to undermine privacy rights, pleading for more refined understandings of public health and wellness. Not content to let detractors suggest they had ill intent, officials implored the public to give the government a chance to prove its good intentions. Some in the department even contended that appeals to privacy might deny economically encumbered residents the opportunity to improve their health. Chamany wrote, "while universal mandatory reporting may include people who do not want their results reported or to receive registry services, a significant proportion of people who would want to be part of the registry and would benefit from its services might not be offered the opportunity for inclusion because of varying practices in obtaining consent unrelated to patients' preferences."[86] The argument reframes diabetes as a systemic harm that needs attention on many fronts, not simply a disease that is the locus of individual management.

Moving from Managing the Epidemic toward Systemic Intervention

Even a perfunctory glimpse at the debate surrounding New York City's registry will provoke discussions about bureaucratic oversight, regulation of the body, and our cultural obsession with averages. The state is unequivocally and unapologetically intruding in the quotidian lives of people in the name of keeping the polis healthy. And yet, if it is true that roughly 8 percent of the US population has diabetes, the more pressing question to ask might be: Are registries, such as those in NYC, a necessity in an age of burgeoning chronic disease? DOHMH has a fluid understanding of the structural dispositions of diabetes, and the city has been tapping into various public works programs and health initiatives to accomplish their goals. Further, when 10–12 percent of our national healthcare budget is now consumed by diabetes care, it is difficult to maintain that this is a wholly private disease.[87]

By taking a broader look at the "epidemic," diabetes can be attacked at its foundations—but only with vigorous resolve. When health departments attempt to survey the cityscape, they do not discern individual bodies, but swaths of residents who share a common struggle with a chronic condition. This is not to deny that the cause and development of diabetes may have distinct qualities across populations, especially as they relate to geography, ethnicity, and socioeconomic status. Still, officials can use these techniques to attest to neighborhoods overridden with fast food and no grocery stores, as is the case in many neighborhoods in cities ranging from Detroit to Atlanta. They might reconceptualize the very idea of "resources" to help those whose social conditions, and not contrived projections of "personal choice," shackle them. Importantly, state and city governments must be careful to assess how local customs, practices, and economic systems impact their messages, lest they end up with ineffectual mechanisms that fail to account for people's everyday lives and initiate no change at all.[88] In that sense, terms such as "epidemic" are but a starting point for government agencies to implement policy measures that might transform the lives of its residents.

To be sure, a degree of uncertainty about the effectiveness of the registry will remain for some time to come. DOHMH runs the risk that the program will fail, or be underfunded, or met with legal hostility. The letters sent to patients, for example, were found to have a clinically nonsignificant influence on A1C scores. Still, the agency continues to avoid the institutionally perilous habit of sliding back into a language that emphasizes personal responsibility and lifestyle choices. The reconfiguring of diabetes as a disease to be communally challenged has not yet been rhetorically palpable for the city and the frame of epidemic may yet be ineffective. Diabetes is an expensive disease, and the real test of this enterprise will come in its ability to continue offering services to residents. Diana Berger, the medical director of the New York City Diabetes Prevention and Control Program, explained that they "wanted to make sure that this was more than just surveillance . . . [and] to design an intervention that would have impact . . . on quality of life."[89] Notably, despite the ubiquitous presence of the tropes "privacy" and "epidemics" in discussions of the registry, the language of personal management continuously resurfaced in disquieting forms. One doctor who supports the idea suggested "that 'an informed and activated patient' is needed, in combination with a coordinated healthcare system." Still, they acknowledged, "we all know this rarely happens." Berger attributed this failure to "rushed practitioners, a lack of coordinated care and active follow-up, and inadequate self-management training for patients."[90]

The state's nuancing of the operation as it evolves must be monitored closely to ensure that the complications faced by those with diabetes are truly understood. In defending the program two public health officials wrote, "Either doctors aren't sharing . . . information with their patients, or they're sharing it and their patients aren't understanding it, or they're sharing it and the patients forget."[91] This three-pronged analysis of life with diabetes is completely centered on the relationship patients have with doctors, mirroring the problematic arguments made by privacy advocates. Certainly, all of these claims may be accurate, but they overlook the point that sometimes people with diabetes are simply drained emotionally by their disease. Sometimes the struggles of everyday life prevent those affected by the disease from focusing on serious medical issues occurring below the surface of the skin. And sometimes the emphasis on management is overbearing and simple-minded.

Rather than stress liberal notions of individual responsibility and financial autonomy, the project can mobilize civic leadership for encountering the disease. DOHMH underscores this in its report, looking to myriad social, cultural, and fiscal resources. According to Chamany, "To promote the self-management of diabetes, the department offers providers additional tools to distribute to patients, such as glucose meters and strips, blood pressure–monitoring cuffs for home use, and free one-year memberships to Department of Parks and Recreation centers."[92] Even progressive measures like the recreation memberships come with their own drawbacks in a city haunted by long winters and geographic obstacles: The memberships assume people can take the time to exercise, have transportation to access it, and the psychological support to succeed. Even with government aid, there are degrees of personal responsibility always inherently at work and those discourses must be carefully engaged. DOHMH is currently using registry data to raise community awareness of diabetes in areas where rates are notably high, to develop programs that focus on the burden of glucose control, and to assist in the placement of community health workers and farmer's markets.

Despite these limitations, the city's efforts may well be worth the fight, especially when measured against the grim realities of diabetes care in many parts of the country. The tools provided by DOHMH, including some forms of health care, make this initiative revelatory. It initially enlisted the support of the New York City Health and Hospitals Corporation, which is a $5.4 billion "public benefit corporation and the largest municipal hospital and health care system in the United States." The network includes "eleven acute care hospitals, six large diagnostic and treatment centers, and eighty community clinics serving nearly 50,000 patients with diabetes."[93] All limits aside, our culture's current path is decidedly not working for those who are economically disadvantaged and living with the condition. DOHMH's advocacy is worth the effort so long as patients are protected from egregious harms.

Although there was some initial outrage toward the program, DOHMH has received little resistance to the registry. Since its implementation, about 90 percent of all labs are participating in the initiative. Most doctors, it would seem, did not flinch at the idea of New York City collecting this data. Physicians have become accustomed to intrusion by third-party managed "care" organizations, and this endeavor likely appears less sinister than HMOs that have wreaked havoc in their hospitals. Since DOHMH had no plans to penalize doctors who treated patients with consistently high blood sugar or to publicly identify those who did, the risks for participating physicians are slight.[94] Indeed, it was always thought that doctors working with less advantaged populations would be confronted with people who had higher A1C levels. City officials would be wise to continue expanding the network of providers that aid socio-economically depressed residents, and they appear to be making good progress on that front as of this writing.

The success of the NYC registry is dependent on the system's ability not only to medically support patients, but also to alter attitudes about diabetes that focus exclusively on self-sovereignty. Currently, both privacy advocates and metaphors emphasizing epidemics do little to shift attitudes that would promote social change. The former renders the disease back to the sector of the individual, doing little to explore the worlds in which New Yorkers live. The latter seeks transformation, even if it lacks a nuanced semiotics for more fully contending with diabetes on its own terms. Then again, there is no reason that we cannot have both an emphasis on privacy and a commitment to making diabetes a public disease free of stigma. But this requires an imagining of the individual as more than a person managing disease on their own—it demands vision on a scale that can come only with a broad understanding of the world occupied by people with diabetes. Tomes reminds us that reformers have long advocated the civic value of public health strategies and that such approaches are effective as long as illness affects people indiscriminately. However, "if a disease affects only some segments of society, especially those already stigmatized for other reasons, its prevention potentially arouses far more hostility and conflict."[95]

People with diabetes and those who support them must continue to be outspoken about treatment modalities supported by public resources. Too many of those living with uncontrolled blood sugars cannot economically, emotionally, or medically manage the disease on their own. People living with HIV/AIDS were able to garner support for a balance between their privacy and their health after long struggles with the medical community and the government. There is a lesson to be learned from the exigency that was sparked by HIV/AIDS activists and the successes they built upon. Those with diabetes are not always as organized as other communities marked by disease, likely because of the lack of urgency that accompanies the condition. This organizing need not exclude doctors, many of whom have a fluid understanding of diabetes's unusual interpersonal and political contours. After all, "Providers caring for 83 percent of patients with elevated A1C tests in the department's South Bronx pilot . . . requested the patient letter service."[96] The lack of organization on the part of local diabetes advocacy groups might also inadvertently further notions of privacy because there are few groups, save the JDRF and the ADA, dedicated to structural changes that would enhance quality of life. To avoid being turned into infantile citizens who must keep their disease private or be seen as mere bodies in public health's vectors, citizens in the rhetorical epidemic must develop a new way of approaching this most chronic of conditions.[97]

New York City Limits: An Addendum

Arguing that the epidemic frame can further progressive purposes in particular situations does not suggest that the trope always serves noble, or even transparently ethical, ends. The utilization of "epidemic," like all symbols, is sometimes beneficial to the project of public health and is sometimes appropriated in ways that will raise eyebrows. In January 2012, representatives at DOHMH stretched the limits of permissibility when they unveiled a controversial ad campaign intended to shock the city's residents. The ad, which was posted throughout the city's cavernous subway system, was part of a contentious effort by then-mayor Michael Bloomberg's administration to raise awareness about the consequences of drinking large quantities of sugary drinks. The municipality introduced a policy that limited the size of such drinks to 16 ounces in restaurants around the five boroughs. The push to curtail soda intake drew the ire of New York's inhabitants, the beverage industry, and a host of political pundits who saw the campaign as government interference run amok. The policy was blocked by at least two courts and never implemented but remains a fierce topic of debate among those who hold

TROUBLED INTERVENTIONS | 169

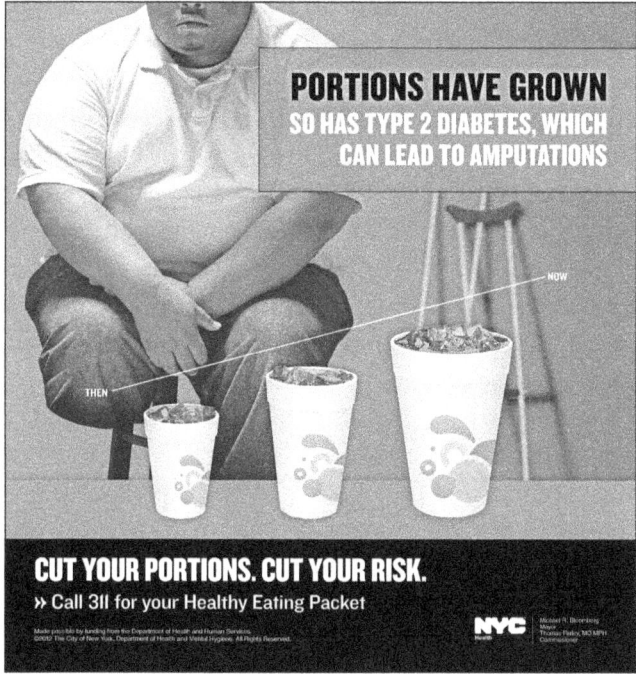

Figure 5.1. NYC DOHMH PSA. New York City Department of Health and Mental Hygiene.

divergent views about the role of institutional intervention and the right of people to be left alone.

The ad in question featured an overweight African American man seated on a stool with an amputated leg. The man is wearing dark pants and a light-colored polo, but the ad's lighting renders everything gray and has the effect of making the picture look spectacularly still. The man's body is visually arresting and the contrast from the grayscale construes his pose as strikingly somber. The amputated leg is on the left side of the frame and a pair of crutches is propped next to the man on the right. A bright red box overlays the top right portion of the ad and contains prose that reads:

> Portions have grown
> So has type-two diabetes, which
> Can lead to amputations

The ad also features three Styrofoam cups, each growing in size from left to right, which are photoshopped in front of the amputee. A superimposed line starting just before the smallest sized cup and placed in the center of the amputated leg reads "Then" and progresses on an angle past the largest cup, which reads "Now." In this way, the ad presents a bit of a temporal incongruity, resting the smallest serving size from days gone by in the center of the amputated leg, but the body with the missing limb is situated in the here and now. Still, the ad's intent is clear enough—portion sizes have grown gluttonous and the people consuming them have followed in kind. At the bottom of the frame the PSA also invites viewers to contact the agency for help managing portion size: "Cut Your Portions, Cut Your Risk. Call 311 for Your Healthy Eating Packet."

The choice to feature an amputated leg in a PSA was made more controversial by the fact that the missing limb was photoshopped. Rather than use an actual person who had lost a leg to diabetes (an uncommon occurrence—foot amputation is much more likely), the agency utilized an able-bodied actor and digitally removed the limb. This ignited a surge of criticism from organizations such as the American Beverage Association, which stood in opposition to the reforms. They grumbled, "This is another example of the 'What can we get away with?' approach that shapes these tax-payer funded ad campaigns."[98] A commentator for *Advertising Age* called it "lazy," "cheap," and "silly," but also relayed that no one was going to lose any sleep over the spot.[99] Not to be dismissed, DOHMH shot back by invoking the epidemic frame:

> When science tells us that smoking does not cause lung cancer or that obesity is not driving an *epidemic* of Type 2 diabetes, we will stop depicting those facts in ads . . . Until then we are going to accurately convey the facts in our advertising—advertising that has helped to successfully reduce smoking in New York City to a historic low of 14 percent, saving thousands of lives.[100]

Representatives from DOHMH argued that such tactics were essential to combating corporations and advertisers who pushed unhealthy products on consumers, often by employing attractive, healthy-looking actors. "Sometimes we use individuals who are suffering from the particular disease; other times we have to use actors . . . We might stop using actors in our ads if the food industry stops using actors in theirs."[101] The "any means necessary" strategy was forwarded with unapologetic bravado. Sadly, it was also produced without thinking through the various ways such an ad might make people with diabetes feel worse about themselves. Fear appeals hold a precarious place in health campaigns. Sometimes they have the desired effect of motivating people to action but can just as easily inspire dissociative tendencies or feelings of despair and helplessness when messages instantiate guilt or shame.

Although the amputated leg generated ample attention, it is significant that the man's face is not fully visible in the photo. What we see of actor Cleo Berry is only from the nose down. His eyes are missing, situating him as an object to be looked at, not a subject who can look back or one who can take action to resolve what ails him. If the eyes are the window to the soul, they are missing, just like his pictorial leg. The short sleeves accentuate Berry's race, an important marker in a PSA that is produced in drab colors. This positioning of the black body as an object for analysis, observation, and treatment reverberates with a history of science looking at black bodies as problems necessitating solutions and not residents who have a moral right to receive support. Unable to constrain his consumption, he is rendered disabled, with fewer opportunities to unburden himself of the ailments he is digitally bequeathed. This questionable ad, clouded by an ableist sensibility and underscored with a racialized projection of disease, does much in the way of shocking viewers and little to educate them. The PSA is also reminiscent of the photo I examined in the introductory chapter, which featured an African American woman walking with a cane and whose head is cropped out of the picture. Like that widely circulated image, this shot illustrates the problematic communion of race, disability, and chronic disease. This condensed metaphor for the diabetes epidemic is at once dingy and spectacular, both highly stylized and resoundingly ordinary. And for all these reasons, the use of this photo by a public health department should offer us pause.

New York City's diabetes registry is groundbreaking for reasons that have nothing to do with shock value or the potential for public spectacle. Rather, it is a banal tool of bureaucracy that performs imperative labor and provides essential resources to those residents most in need. The utilization of "epidemic" as a trope for government mobilization in DOHMH's rhetoric serves the laudable goal of initiating a collective conversation about diabetes by reaching out to those who might be isolated by feelings of shame and stigma or who might not have the means to manage the disease. In contrast, the agency here employed figurations of the "epidemic" to justify suspicious outreach practices and was rightfully reprimanded for a momentary ethical lapse. Nonetheless, the uptake of the trope of "epidemic" need not be construed as dubious in all instances. In the context of a chronic condition that is savaging countless people, the municipality can rein in the effects of diabetes by being a partner that extols the promise of institutional intervention and the necessity of collective action.

6

Cyborg Dreams

In 2013, the National Museum of American History in Washington, DC curated an exhibit called "The Birth of Biotech." The display celebrated the dawn of genetic engineering in the 1970s and the cultural significance of recombinant pharmaceuticals in the context of US national identity. Lauding the innovation of recombinant DNA, a technique that permits scientists to extract DNA from two sources and then fuse them together, continued a Smithsonian tradition of consecrating scientific progress as an exceptional component of the nation's character. The colorful museum labels captioning the gallery tell visitors that this particular breakthrough was the result of both "cutting-edge science and high-risk investment," highlighting the centrality of venture capitalism even as it omits institutions, such as public universities, that were foundational to such research. The introduction of mass-produced recombinant DNA is presented as a hallmark of American ingenuity, the dexterity of free enterprise, and the ongoing project of pioneering vanguard technologies. Most important for the purposes of this book is the exhibit's case study, the firstborn child of the marriage between genetic engineering and capitalism: human insulin.

The offspring metaphor is used purposefully here, in part because the most striking feature of the display is a large black and white photo of a young boy giving himself an insulin injection. The image is one of the few objects in the exhibit not donated by Genentech, the corporation being extolled by the museum.[1] As this book has illustrated, the visual trope of the child is represented repeatedly in diabetes history. The recurring presence of children with diabetes served as a testament to the resurrection effects of insulin in "before and after" photos of patients in the 1920s and continues to structure media coverage of organizations such as the JDRF. The image of the anonymous boy underscores the value of synthetic human insulin as part of the long tradition of keeping children alive and with them the hopes and dreams of the nation's

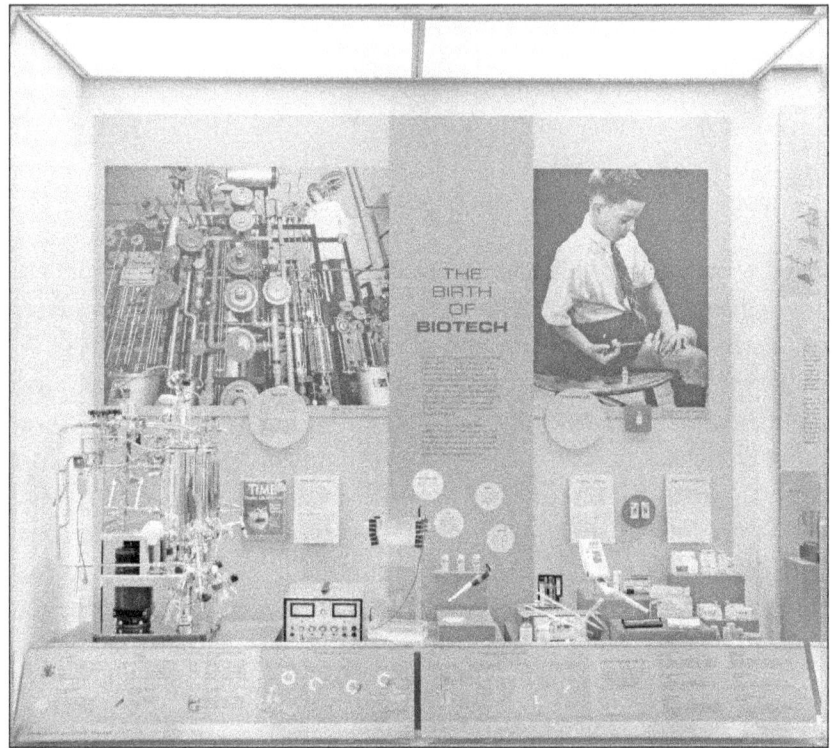

Figure 6.1. "The Birth of Biotech," Archives Center, National Museum of American History, Smithsonian Institution.

future. The child in question is white, has a fresh crew cut, and is dressed in a light-colored shirt and dark shorts with what appears to be a plaid tie. He is seated in profile to the viewer as he injects himself with insulin in his exposed right leg. The photo is striking not only because of its stark black and white contrast, but also because the syringe and the needle look unusually large against his body. His clean-cut appearance and relatively diminutive size make the medical instrument seem invasive, if not visually pain-inducing, for visitors to the site. The picture is also unusually staged in the display. To start, the object label beneath the photo instructs viewers that this is a snapshot from the 1950s or 1960s, well before the advent of recombinant DNA technologies. The child is a metonym for the inspired, if flawed, history of diabetes innovation just as much as he is an involuntary champion for the biogenetics being lionized. Further, the picture's placement in the mnemoscape produces an incongruity that is noteworthy in a feature focused on the effects of science. The image of the boy is situated to the right of a large color photo of a Willy Wonka-esque machine from the early 1980s that was used in the genetic engineering process. Although the "biotech" segment of the display is contained entirely to the left side of the case and the "history of insulin" portion to the right (separated by a red, elongated placard that reads "The Birth of Biotech"), the positioning of the images suggest a cause and effect movement from synthetic human insulin to self-care that is undermined by both the time line of discovery and the color schemes of the photos. The spectacular representation of insulin's reproduction on the left side of the display is assuredly not the same substance being used by the boy to its right. Until the early 1980s, animal-based insulins, which were extracted from the pancreases of cows and pigs, were the only options available to people with diabetes. The young boy is most certainly using a bovine- or porcine-based insulin. Of course, one need not read these images sequentially to appreciate the full effect of their presentation. In fact, the distribution of the photos can be read as rhetorically consequential if we privilege the movement of technology *into* the human body and situate the past not as nostalgic, but with the relief that one era has waned and another has arrived. The antiquated, animal-based insulin contained in the obtrusive syringe held against the child's leg has been replaced by modernistic manufactured "human" analogue insulin and enthymematically imbues this technology with affectively positive associations.[2]

Despite the revolutionary advancement of recombinant DNA at the time, the curators acknowledge that anxieties and risks pervade its storied conception. They note that gene splicing "generated reactions ranging from fear of its potential risks to eager anticipation of its potential benefits." These historical asterisks are not without precedent. The dialectic between the bold necessity of scientific progress and the hesitations it produces is a constant feature of diabetes's biography and quietly underscores the exhibit.[3] A time line in the display detailing the tools used for diabetes management relays that prior to "the introduction of disposable syringes, needles had to be regularly sterilized and sharpened" before use, yet another muted inducement of pain that indirectly communicates the benefits of contemporary medicine. The words "purification" and "purify" appear in descriptive remarks to exalt the advantages of synthetic insulin, even as there is little indication that genetically inspired insulins were safer or more effective than their animal-based corollaries, a debate that will be discussed later in the chapter. The curator marginalia also subtly intermixes, if not outright confuses, type 1 and type 2 diabetes by discussing "unhealthy changes in lifestyle and eating habits," even as they visually deploy the young boy to denote the benefactors of insulin therapy, likely for people with type 1. The idea of risk murmurs throughout the piece: in the investments being made in genetic engineering, the hesitations of citizens about the ramifications of biogenetic techniques, the "impurity" of older insulin extracts, and the subsiding of danger thanks to the advent of new technologies. But even as risk and apprehension lurk, progress, we are told, has assuredly won the day.

The exhibit's unusual mediation of temporality, asking audiences in the second decade of the new millennium to weigh the advancements of late-twentieth-century technology against a single shot (medicinal and photographic) taken decades earlier, illustrates the scientific mythos of diabetes technology and hints at the unease that frequently underlines such progress. Scholars have long noted the ideological commitments embedded in terms such as "progress," particularly as they materialize in rhetorics of American exceptionalism. Richard Weaver went so far as to call "progress" America's most potent god term, a word that is not only revered but one that establishes relations among other expressions.[4] The memory practices instigated by the display, in the context of a still incurable disease, communicate an ongoing faith placed in technological advancements and the ways developments in diabetes care continue to foster both hope and apprehension. As the museum's director John Gray commented, "The story of biotechnology inspires the type of critical and inventive thinking that has allowed Americans to excel in emerging technologies throughout the nation's history . . . The museum helps visitors to understand these past advances as a foundation for future progress."[5] In an era where insulin pens and pumps command the market, and scientists and advocates eye artificial pancreases and decidedly futuristic devices such as contact lenses equipped with microchips to gauge glucose levels, the road ahead seems as promising as ever for those who can afford the high cost of being ill. Diabetes is a chronic condition, one marked by its relationship to time (*chronos*), and technology functions to alleviate the unknowns that dwell in one's future. In some ways the temporal frame of the future has been a constant companion to the metaphors explored in each chapter of this book, accentuating attitudes about the supposed ease of managing health, the certainty of death, the longevity made possible by highly informed agentic agents, and the promise of communal well-being. This chapter provides a synthesis to those fluid and multilayered tropes, not attempting to reconcile their sometimes-contradictory materializations but thinking through the cultural and rhetorical consequences of their byzantine circulation in everyday life.

Rhetoric that emboldens the promise of technology can simultaneously inspire hope, triumph, struggle, and the just-out-of-reach capacity of science to radically reconfigure lives. This was true when insulin was championed as a gateway to a cure in the early 1920s. It was true when the biotechnologies featured at the Smithsonian were manufactured in the early 1980s. It remains true today as people with diabetes invest their energies and dreams into the prospects of a self-sustaining digitized organ like the artificial pancreas. At each interval there have been achievements to applaud and reasons to pause. As people with diabetes continue to adopt machinist apparatuses to enhance and prolong life, the prospects and shortcomings of management discourses continue to demand scrutiny, provoking questions about the frameworks guiding public rhetorics, the boundlessness of scientific enterprise, and the affordability of technological innovation.

Cyborg Manifestations

The associations outlined among biologics, genetic informatics, and the corporate colonization of the body in the Smithsonian's memorializing harkens back to themes engaged by Donna Haraway in her widely read "cyborg manifesto." It may seem cliché to begin a chapter about the communion of organisms and machines with Haraway's infamous musings about the blurred lines between individuals and technology. But it also feels like academic malpractice to start anywhere else. The "human" insulin being celebrated in the exhibit, for example, is a misnomer because it is not actually "human," but a synthetic substance grown using bacteria or yeast. In Haraway's words, "we are all chimeras, theorized and fabricated hybrids of machine and organism; in short, we are cyborgs. The cyborg is our ontology; it gives us our politics."[6] Haraway's essay has been referred to as "theoretical science fiction" but it laudably (and ambitiously) sought to subvert taxonomies that reproduce and reify modes of domination by identifying technological shifts that challenge power structures maintained through antagonistic dualisms (such as mind/body, man/woman, and human/machine).[7] Haraway argues that social relations are best contemplated outside the dichotomous tendencies of Western thought and that there is pleasure in the confusion of boundaries and responsibility in their construction.[8] In this way, the figure of the cyborg is not a fanciful creature in a distant time or place, nor is it sequestered to the pages of science fiction.[9] Rather, it is a heuristic for thinking politics anew. We are all, to some extent, a product of and in the process of becoming cyborg.[10] If literary theorist Kenneth Burke told us that we are separated from our natural condition by tools of our own making, a "sheer animality" that was abandoned with the adoption of symbol systems, Haraway contends that such natural conditions are patently inconceivable.[11] We are bound inextricably to the technologies that situate us as inherently cultural. As Tom Foster surmises, "technology no longer plays a dialectical role as the Other of humanity; instead, that otherness exists within the 'human,' thereby denaturalizing the assumptions about the relation between body and cultural identity."[12] Critics who embrace the potential of Haraway's cyborg myth tend to treat with great suspicion those who proclaim a return to a "natural" or essential identity.[13] This certainly rings true for people with disabilities and those struggling with disease and illness, as the very idea of a "natural" state can be tantamount to a death sentence.

Haraway contended that three chimeric evolutions have transformed human identity: the blurring of boundaries among humans and animals, machines and bodies, and the physical and non-physical. The history of diabetes technology finds that a case could be made for any of these obscured lines, but I focus attention primarily on the second, with some reference to the third, in this chapter. Haraway places the development of cyborg consciousness somewhere between the late nineteenth century and the 1930s, enveloping the time that insulin was discovered in 1922.[14] In what might be considered a chance encounter, her manifesto was published just months after recombinant DNA was approved by the FDA, and that innovation is often referred to, appropriately, as "chimeric DNA." Haraway's cyborg sensibility escorts diabetes technology and its human dependents in much the same way it does her allusions to militaristic or scientific innovation. The modern reliance on glucose monitors, insulin pens, and pumps suggests a subject constituted explicitly by quotidian engagements with technology. The sheer amount of data provided by monitors and pumps underscores the relationality of biogenetics and information central to how endocrinologists treat disease, how care is managed, and how people understand their bodies against an imagined medical norm. Sophisticated electrode technologies to read glucose levels actualize the dilapidation between the physical and nonphysical realms of being, acting in concert with the indistinguishable line between machine and organism, to produce a cyborg encounter. If the figure of the cyborg was useful in detailing the fragmented experience of feminist politics in the early 1980s, I believe it continues to be an invaluable perspective for contemplating the negotiation of chronic conditions and technology in the twenty-first century, especially insofar as people with differing kinds of diabetes are often situated against one another in the public sphere.

The cyborg is a particularly instrumental heuristic because it troubles the tendency to partition diabetes as the domain of a sovereign subject on the one hand and as the object of medical regard and technological experimentation on the other. The devices and pharmaceuticals that rein in diabetes's effects are now attached to or circulate within the body on a nearly constant basis: Long-lasting insulins course through the blood 24 hours a day; pumps and continuous glucose monitors (CGMs) are worn not only to work or school, but to bed and in the swimming pool. The body is not a machine in the spirit of the early-twentieth-century metaphor per se, but life apart from these technologies is inconceivable. To separate the person with diabetes from modern medical innovations is to invite their demise. Haraway argues that machines were once marked by a dualism between "materialism and idealism that was settled by a dialectical progeny, called spirit or history, according to taste."[15] This common philosophical schism between the constitution of human consciousness through symbols (idealism) and the "primary substance of all living and non-living things" or "matter" (materialism) hints at our present-day cyborg consciousness: Attempting to achieve the normative ideals of health has become inextricably linked to innovations that combat material disease.[16] The line between human and machine has been dissolved by an integration of the agent who performs diabetes management and their body, which is the scene of treatment.[17] The body of the patient has been melded with technologies that keep them alive, and that communion is the site of medical knowledge.[18] This expertise is not confined to the space of the clinic, but must be continually reenacted by people with diabetes. Haraway's quip that our machines are "disturbingly lively" and people "frighteningly inert" seems especially noteworthy in a discussion about technological horizons and the worries they inaugurate.[19] To be sure, I do not believe that people with diabetes are on the verge of becoming machines in the most literal sense. Too many patients and medical practitioners remain skeptical of the redemption such technologies offer. Rather, I use the blurred line betwixt agent and scene to think through the promise and perils of technology on the diabetic body.

Throughout this book I have argued that the semiosis of diabetes management is not easily reducible to any set of metaphors or tropological figures. The bodies of people with diabetes, their everyday practices, the anxieties that lurk beneath medical and activist endeavors, and the circulation of discourses about the disease all materialize in situated contexts that enliven diabetes as an object of knowledge. Like Haraway, I believe that meaning-making is "the struggle for language and struggle against perfect communication, against the one code that translates all meaning perfectly, the central dogma of phallogocentrism."[20] The power to signify is both the basis of political power and a necessary tool of survival.[21] The tropology of language offers entry into formal systems, which are transformed through tactical acts of resistance. Haraway notes:

> I'm interested in tropes as places where you trip. Tropes are way more than metaphors and metonymies and the narrow orthodox list. Noise is only one figure, one trope that I'm interested in. Tropes are about stutterings, trippings. They are about breakdowns and that's why they are creative. That is why you get somewhere you weren't before, because something didn't work.[22]

The ruptures that enamor Haraway are made possible, in part, by the fissures and failures in technological endeavors. These hiccups in innovation will sometimes maintain the order, sometimes resist it, and still other times perform both simultaneously. Each of these must be "localized in a system architecture whose basic modes of operation are probabilistic" and not overdetermined.[23] Language is the gateway to politics and the cyborg is one figuration for keeping open the utility of critique without resorting to origin stories and essentialized understandings of the self. Or, in this case, any one figuration for making disease intelligible.

The gene splicing performed by Genentech and the insulin pumps worn by people with diabetes approximate how a cyborg identity typically might be conceived—as part human and part machine. But this understanding only captures one dimension of Haraway's manifesto, which is committed to challenging rigid identity categories and advocating for more transformative political affinities. One of Haraway's most widely circulated claims is that politics should divest itself of origin stories and totalizing theories, remaining open to an array of identifications to rethink the future. Her writings give presence to the problematic logics of universals, the limits of narrowed epistemologies, and the promise provided by the dearth of information that humans possess about themselves. I excavate moments in the history of diabetes technology, especially those that conjoin the hopes and anxieties of innovation, to contemplate future trajectories of management rhetoric.

The remainder of this chapter explores the merging of the human and the machine to think through the evolution of diabetes technology. I close this chapter by pondering the ideas of risk and anxiety not as explicitly attached to technology, but the capitalistic impulses that keep such technology out of reach for scores of people. Importantly, what follows is not meant to be a rehearsing of paranoid views of technology. Nor is it meant to be a full account of diabetes breakthroughs. That task has been performed elsewhere with extensive historical detail and to better effect. Rather, I look to the advent of specific innovations to chart a narrative about instrumentality and opportunity, situated action and the prolonged discourse of hope. For Haraway, inhabiting the cyborg is part of "an obligatory worldmaking" that initiates "radical possibilities."[24] I echo Haraway's declaration that "cyborg figurations can continue to do critical work" to imagine culture anew.²⁵ Next I give presence to the blurring of boundaries between medical technology and human bodies before turning more explicitly to management politics to think through the future of diabetes activism and the high cost of staying well.

The Promise and Peril of Diabetes Technology: The Discovery of Insulin

Researchers heralded insulin as one of the most important discoveries of modern medicine when it arrived on the scene in 1922. Doctors and patients alike described it as a "miracle" because of the immediacy of its impact and the transformative effects it had on the bodies of those being treated.²⁶ To say that insulin radically altered the lives of people with diabetes is to understate the full consequences of its introduction. Prior to the arrival of insulin, a person diagnosed at age ten could expect to live no more than three years. Those diagnosed with type 2 diabetes after age sixty generally had about six years before the disease killed them. Chris Feudtner notes in his compelling history of type 1 diabetes that few scientific advancements have been lauded with the mythic "technology ethos" that undergirds the discovery of insulin. Insulin was quickly established as a "medical marvel," to borrow a phrase from Jenell Johnson, because the substance superseded its own medicinal purposes and was rhetorically saturated with conflicting origin stories, debates over purpose, and public acclaim.²⁷ Early testimonials about insulin championed its potency "as a heroic wonder drug to rescue patients, vanquish disease, banish suffering" and alter the scripts of everyday life.²⁸ Keeping with a theme visited repeatedly in this book, one of the unforeseen consequences of insulin's discovery was the "happily-ever-after" account of life with diabetes that circulated widely and that did not accurately reflect the daily realities of management.²⁹ Public narratives extolling the ease of management quickly supplanted the fatalism that characterized medical anecdotes about diabetes treatment, care, and longevity.

The discourse surrounding insulin tended to reiterate a common tale about medical intervention but often eclipsed the hesitation and apprehension among some physicians and their patients. At least since Plato expressed dismay about the potential of writing to displace the robust dialogues that prevailed in his day, new technologies have been repeatedly accused of disintegrating everything from communal bonds to interpersonal intimacy.[30] Even when breakthroughs are embraced and assimilated into the landscape of conventional practice, they are frequently accompanied by so-called revenge effects, those unforeseen consequences of technological progress and development.[31] Insulin was no exception, instigating concern among parents and doctors that children faced novel harms, be it from low blood sugar during the night, or opportunistic infections, or the harmful effects of acidosis.[32] Some doctors worried that patients "would make potentially lethal mistakes" when left to their own devices.[33] In this way insulin was a "precious but flawed miracle."[34] Michael Bliss points out in his detailed history of the discovery of insulin that some doctors were so conservative in their approach that they refused to prescribe it when the substance was introduced.[35]

Perhaps paradoxically, even as the implementation of insulin regimens masked the everyday struggles of diabetes complications, it also gave rise to a lexicon that structured medical understandings of the condition. Flipping through Feudnter's work, we find references to "learning the language of diabetic life," "the grammar of routine," and "narration and creating meaning in life."[36] The promise of insulin simultaneously provided the hope of a prolonged life span but also engendered assumptions that overstated the ease of management. Prior to the discovery of long-lasting, 24-hour insulins, for example, people often planned their daily routines around spikes in insulin that required them to eat at precise intervals following injections. One long-time friend with diabetes told me that when she was diagnosed in 1984, she mixed two insulins and took one shot in the morning, which then peaked twice: once after two hours and then again six hours later (covering breakfast and lunch). She then repeated the routine for dinner and an evening snack. Of course, such a regimen also required one to eat the same amount of food every day and almost always at approximately the same time. Variability is a common feature of most people's lives, but the dictates of management did not always foster the freedoms one might presuppose. Insulin enabled people with diabetes to live longer but also demanded an acute awareness of their bodies and their surroundings. In an era before cell phones, being in a car far from access to food, for example, could be a precarious venture. This is not to say that insulin therapies are without risks today. As recently as 2011, the JDRF warned that one in twenty people with diabetes will die from hypoglycemia.[37] Injecting insulin is a better alternative than death, of course, and I am not trying to suggest otherwise. It is, however, worth noting that fatalism, an agentic agent, and the ease of living with disease all enter the equation when assessing risk. Management is a complicated condensation of discourses that is sometimes easily navigated and at other times difficult to untangle.

The enthusiastic reception of new technologies is omnipresent in diabetes's long history, even when the benefits to patients are questionable. Take the transition from animal-sourced insulins to those made by recombinant DNA technology. The substance was originally culled from the pancreases of cows and pigs, because the strand of amino acids that make up human insulin are remarkably similar to the ones found in those mammals. The extracted insulin was then purified to avoid adverse reactions in a person's body. The advent of biotechnology that enabled synthetic "human" insulin through gene splicing was publicly lauded as a landmark achievement, because it avoided such impurities and it could be readily mass-produced.[38] Dr. Irving L. Spratt, then head of the American Diabetes Association, touted that the new science was "an exciting event in medicine. It demonstrates the melding of intensive research in genetic engineering with complex pharmaceutical production."[39] The excitement seems unusual in retrospect, in large part because the discovery had little effect on the outcomes of patient health. The new creations were no more effective than animal-based insulins common at the time, they cost more, exacerbated the effects of hypoglycemia, and eventually limited consumer choice for people living with diabetes. It is not conspiratorial to speculate that the motive for recombinant DNA insulin was not simply medical, but for revenue-generating purposes. As one source told the *Washington Post*, "If you were diabetic and could buy pig insulin or 'human' insulin at the same price, which would you choose? It's an advertising man's dream."[40] Some commentators surmised that mass-produced insulin might be necessary as diabetes rates climbed because unlimited supplies could be harvested from bacteria, but no evidence exists that increased incidences of diabetes provided the impetus for the technology's genesis.

What is perhaps most astounding in retrospect is the degree to which commercial profit from the innovation was downplayed in the early 1980s. Numerous reports argued that Humulin, the brand name given to "human insulin," would not have a significant impact on manufacturer Eli Lilly's bottom line, in part because the company already owned 85 percent of the market and in part because biogenetics was an expensive undertaking. Securities analysts deduced that the product "is not going to be of commercial significance."[41] Such assertions seemed especially suspect in light of the immense profits Lilly earned when insulin first hit the market in the 1920s.[42] It would be misleading to suggest that there was little public dialogue about cost, profits, and consumer burden when the new insulin was developed, but its promise always seemed to eclipse any potential drawbacks. I'll address the price of insulin at the end of this chapter as one of the most significant issues related to diabetes advocacy today, but suffice it to say for now that a "technobiopower" had emerged in the United States around diabetes technologies. That is, technologies not only functioned to maintain the health of people with diabetes, but also situated bodies in a network of power relations articulated to laborious surveillance and laissez-faire consumerism, demanding an activated patient able to prolong life and maximize profits for corporations.[43] At the very moment that HIV started to occupy the attention of scientists and catalyze activists, people with diabetes emerged as consumers, encouraged to adopt the newest forms of insulin to stave off complications. Fatalism always lurked both inside the body and from external sources and it was up to individual patients to embrace the technological promise of novel discoveries. New innovations promised to delay diabetes's cataclysmic effects, but only insofar as people were willing to subscribe to the high cost of new insulins. The imperative not to "live in the past" was essential to Humulin's branding.

The pressure on people with diabetes to adopt Humulin became prominent almost as soon as recombinant insulins were approved. The "marketer's dream" came to life in both the United States and the United Kingdom, as corporations sought to expand profits and displace other products. This movement is exemplified in an essay published by Jeremy Green and Kevin Riggs in the *New England Journal of Medicine* detailing the absence of generic insulin. The authors reprinted an Eli Lilly advertisement from 1984, which was the year Humulin was made publicly available, alongside their article. Green and Riggs employ the ad to underscore the manufacturer's aggressive marketing techniques and explicit use of emotional appeals. This particular ad is most compelling to me because of the image that accompanies it, one that echoes the Smithsonian photo examined at the start of this chapter. Like the black and white image, this advertisement features a young boy giving himself an insulin shot. As with the boy in the Birth of Biotech exhibit, the child is white and administering the shot himself, save perhaps the aid of a Teddy Bear and a Boba Fett action figure flanking him. Unlike the child discussed earlier, he is shirtless (literally exposed) and situated on a cream-colored couch in what appears to be a living room. The picture is warm, with a clear view of a radiator, a multicolored rug, a wicker basket, and flowered curtains. The boy's shoes are strewn on the floor, clearly indicating that he is at home. The text immediately beneath the boy's picture reads, "He's four years old. And already he's living in the past." If the JDRF utilized fatalism to ally lawmakers in their search for a cure, then the makers of Humulin embraced it as a scare tactic to constitute a new consumer subject. The visualization of the private sphere communicates security, warmth, and ease in the ad. But there is also a danger in the house—a past to which this boy is barely privy but one that assuredly determines his future. Humulin must be taken to save his life.

If enthusiasm marks the public transcript of diabetes technologies, the hidden transcript is often one of suspicion, hesitation, and doubt, especially for many people with diabetes who must navigate management's omnipresent demands. This on-the-ground recalcitrance indicates occasions of tropological tripping, ways in which the drawbacks of progress can be identified and carefully scrutinized. For example, in the early 1980s the FDA warned that any change in insulin regimens should be "made cautiously and under medical supervision."[44] The transition from animal-based insulins to synthetic human insulin proved challenging for scores of people who had been using the former for decades. In Britain, more than 15,000 people were said to be at risk from the new insulins, with thousands of people reporting that they were passing out from hypoglycemia without warning and many of those same patients telling doctors that they were suffering convulsions and memory loss.[45] These experiences were collected in the early 1990s but suppressed by the British Diabetes Association for six years because they found the report to be "too alarmist." To quell these fears in the United States, Eli Lilly initially encouraged a phased introduction of the medicine to the

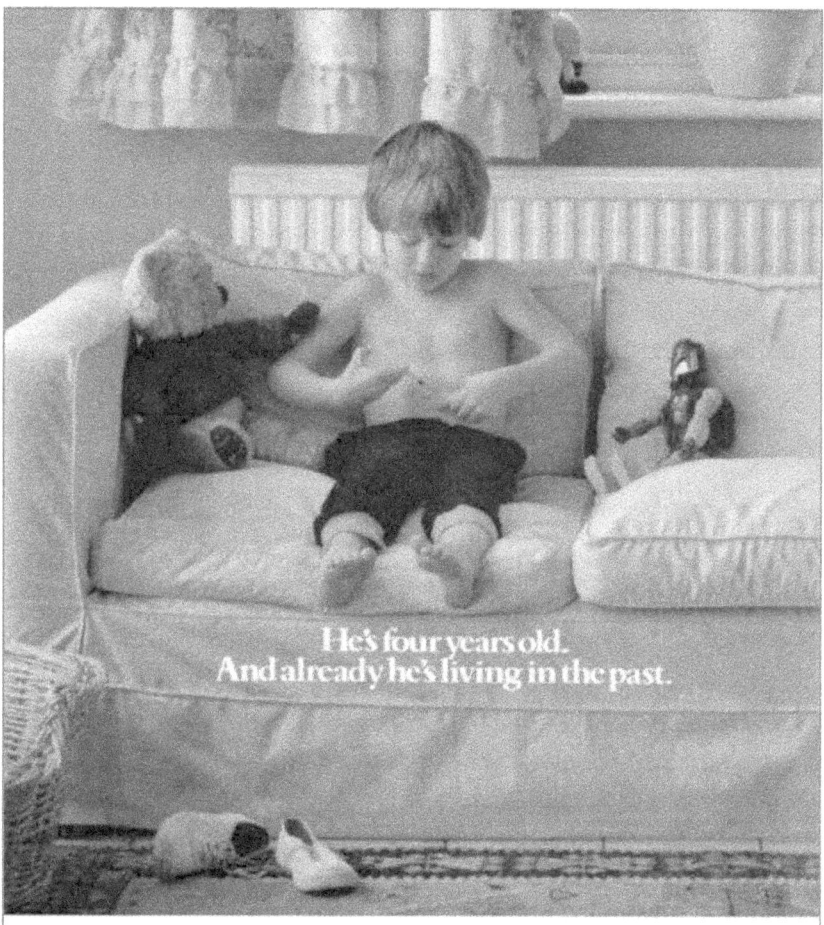

Figure 6.2. Humulin Ad. © Copyright Eli Lilly and Company. All Rights Reserved. Photo courtesy of Eli Lilly and Company Archives.

public before making it commercially available. Innovation can be transformative, but its stumbles remain equally disconcerting in demarcating who is profiting from intervention, who is being left open to risk, and how those most implicated in change maintain presence in a system that insists on the slow march of progress.

This is not to say that all medical practitioners are skeptical of newly developed technologies, including the continued refinement of engineered insulin analogs. Even as costs have continued to skyrocket, the ongoing purification of insulin has proven to make life more livable for countless people who have diabetes. Insulin made from "designer microorganisms" tends to incite fewer allergic reactions and is absorbed better than previously used animal-based insulins.[46] In some instances, animal-based insulins slowly became less effective than genetically modified ones. This is to say nothing of the ethical questions that arise from using animal parts to craft such medicines. Porcine and bovine insulins were originally developed from the discarded pancreases of pigs and cows slaughtered by the meat industry. Insulin derived from pork and beef is virtually identical to that of people, but enormous numbers of animals were required to manufacture small amounts of the substance. Prior to the development of biotechnologies, it took roughly two tons of pig pancreases just to extract eight ounces of purified insulin. Today's insulins allow users to manipulate how quickly insulin is absorbed into the system, and hence permit greater options for blood sugar control, even if they are more expensive and sometimes come with a learning curve. Clearly, they also foster a more environmentally sustainable practice that is conscious of other living animals.

The history of scientific advancement is frequently shadowed by the fears and anxieties accompanying new technologies. Inventions meant to better the human experience are regularly punctuated by misgivings about cultural changes in the present and the implications of those developments for the future. Even as innovation is supposed to make life more manageable, exchanges about technology are often replete with nostalgia for times that were supposedly simpler, kinder, and more personable. These jitters are part and parcel of technological evolution and can be found in everything from social media memes to memorials dedicated to modernization and the scientific frontier.[47] Diabetes technology is no exception, though anxiety is not necessarily contained to one sphere. Sometimes apprehension is found in the concerns of practitioners who believe patients move too quickly to adopt technology for the wrong reasons. At other times people with diabetes appear suspicious of new medicines that might interrupt routines or contribute to multinational corporate profiteering. The dialectical tension between the necessity of medical intervention to sustain health and the hesitation those developments initiate are especially pronounced in considerations of new devices such as insulin pumps and the still developing artificial pancreas.

From Pumps to Pancreases and Beyond: The Continued Evolution

The advent of the insulin pump is one marked by the promise of unending information and amplified self-awareness every bit as it is the mechanical delivery of medicine. An insulin pump is a small, computerized device about the size of a cell phone that delivers insulin to the body, usually through the use of tubing and a catheter. Unlike individual shots, pumps provide a constant stream of insulin around the clock.[48] Many of the devices now utilize a continuous glucose monitor (CGM), which takes blood sugar readings throughout the day and offers feedback about the amount of insulin required to normalize blood sugars. Insulin pump manufacturers such as Medtronic maintain that their devices are wildly advantageous and reduce complications to the kidneys, the cardiovascular and nervous systems, and the eyes.[49] Their marketing materials also contend that pumps require 90 percent fewer shots, even as most people recognize the trade-off of having one or two catheters inserted perpetually into their skin. Pumps can facilitate diverse kinds of information, including trends in blood sugar and the amount of insulin needed for different foods. The unfettered supply of data provided by pumps may very well constitute them as the example par excellence of cyborg life. Past devices, such as the one developed by Arnold Kadish in the early 1960s, aspired to give people with diabetes the ability to control their disease effortlessly but focused largely on maintaining health in the moment, as the technology to process information about sugars and adjust the self accordingly did not yet exist. Kadish's futuristic-looking machine reflected the scientific fetishization of the period, literally having the appearance of a jetpack, but its daunting size prohibited it from ever appearing on the market. Today's pumps are less obtrusive and have become especially popular for their convenience, though there are a host of reasons to explain their popularity that are not easily reduced to technological determinism. The incorporation of the insulin pump into management regimens reflects a desire for ever more information, feelings of personal sovereignty and mobility, and an ability to be public while maintaining privacy. In this way insulin pumps are culturally resonant with smart phones. Insulin pumps not only keep the body in motion, they align well with contemporary understandings of the self, ones that are grounded in cosmopolitan ideals of community and individuality.

The ability to self-surveil is not without its consequences and requires a reiteration of self-sustaining rituals in order to maintain the benefits of technological innovations. Medtronic cautions that there are numerous limitations associated with the pump and asserts that its use is not recommended for people unwilling to perform a minimum of four blood glucose tests a day, stay in close contact with a physician, and be relentlessly vigilant. The company is quick to offer warnings about the dangers of hyperglycemia if insulin is interrupted, the ensuing threat of diabetic ketoacidosis (DKA), and note that stress and illness can increase the chances of glucose irregularities. Further, the company provides warnings about the need to change infusion sites to avoid the buildup of scar tissue that can interrupt the delivery of insulin and the potential for infections, and also recommends carrying an "emergency kit" of supplies for the pump *and* additional forms of insulins and syringes in the event the device malfunctions. CGM readings can also be concerning because they read glucose levels on a delay. As one source noted, it "takes glucose around 5–10 minutes to move from blood into tissue fluid, or back, so the CGMS measures lag behind what's really happening in your blood if things are changing rapidly."[50] In what might sound like something out of a spy thriller, many people have raised concerns about information privacy and the potential hacking of insulin pumps.[51] More recently, diabetes advocates have called for manufacturers to share information about malfunctioning pumps with researchers.[52] It is difficult to approximate how often pumps break down, but it is estimated that one in four people using a pump for a year experiences pump failure.[53] This is not to say that a pump is any less advantageous than other forms of management, but public discourse tends to accentuate its technological revelations, the ease of treatment it affords, and the privacy it engenders. Nonetheless, fatalism shades the literature about the pump, which demands an agentic agent who can bring the technology's potential to fruition.

The blurring of agent and machine instigates quandaries about the functionality of management devices and the extent to which technological interventions can actually bring sugar numbers closer to "normal" range. As one nurse practitioner told me, pumps are but a tool for managing diabetes, not a solution to its many problems. Pump technology has innumerable advantages but has also produced a disquieting discourse among some medical providers that people will give themselves over to the machines unreflexively, not acting with discernable personal agency, but with a casual attitude that throws to the wind a rigorous approach to care. The internet abounds with materials that relay these anxious sentiments, but generally under innocuous headings such as, "Who Should Go on an Insulin Pump?" and "Is the Insulin Pump Right for You?" A closer look finds declarations that the patient must "stay motivated," that "commitment is required," and that "psychological readiness and psychological needs vary with individuals." On a practical level, such concerns are not entirely unwarranted. How does one strike a balance between the patterns and ratios that guide the devices with commonsense readings of the body in situ that most people with diabetes depend on as survival skills? How does one reconcile that a pump can measure insulin at a microscopic level *and* that it increases the chances for DKA? What does it mean to harmonize the techne of diabetes management with the prudence gleaned from everyday experiences living with the disease? More than ever before, pump technology requires the patient to perform clinical expertise.

Interestingly, CGMs appear to be having a greater impact on the regulation of blood sugars than are insulin pump technologies. Insulin pumps do not necessarily allow for additional control—they merely deliver insulin. CGMs, however, offer near immediate data to users and in the process raise awareness of A1C levels. Even as I was revising this chapter, CGMs were evolving at a tremendous clip. Many CGMs have required users to prick their fingers at least twice a day to calibrate them.

As of the completion of this chapter, several of these devices now come pre-calibrated in the factory. Still, there are limitations to the quality of life provided by any technology. My own endocrinologist has suggested that a number of studies currently being conducted about CGMs focus on the quality of life they provide to patients. Some manufacturers do not permit low blood glucose alarms to be turned off during the night, which means these devices often keep people awake and interrupt the potential to rest. This is true even when sugars are not dangerously low. Self-surveillance can produce feelings of ambivalence and malaise, even when the outcomes are generally favorable from a clinical perspective.

The natural heir to the insulin pump is the artificial pancreas, a closed-loop system that also uses an insulin pump and a CGM to regulate the body's blood sugars. The daunting task of how to incorporate the delivery of glucose and insulin into the body concurrently has not come easily and as of today there is no device with the distinction of being an "artificial pancreas" in the most literal sense. The promise of this ever-elusive faux organ was bolstered in 2016 when the FDA approved a hybrid closed-loop system for automating insulin dosage to manage blood sugars.[54] Scientists hailed it as a "game changer" and enthusiasm for the device was trumpeted by activist organizations, by social media users, and by the national press corps. Reaction to the technology had been especially jubilant because clinical trial participants experienced no severe hypoglycemic episodes, nor did any of the 124 people using the device suffer from ketoacidosis. One user reported, "I'm spending a lot less time worrying about [diabetes] and managing it. I can just look at the pump and see what my blood sugar is at any time, and it pretty much takes care of the ongoing controlling of it."[55] This man's words impart the cybernetic dreams of relinquishing personal responsibility to the machine, but also affirm some fears among medical practitioners—technology is supposed to enhance consciousness, not erode it. The trial found that the pumps kept people in their desired sugar ranges 73.4 percent of the time versus 67.8 percent without the system.[56] The JDRF was one of the many partners to champion the device, and as enthusiastic as their press release was, they made sure to note that these machines were meant to "accelerate ways to a cure" and not act as a stop-gap.[57] Importantly, the Medtronic device was approved only for people with type 1 diabetes who are older than fourteen years of age. The age requirement signals the need for a sentient actor who can maintain the burdensome balance of applying broad principles to complex situations and not a patient who will abdicate control.

The public transcript of triumph and enthusiasm accompanying this newfangled technology is unsurprising when we view it against the celebratory history of diabetes technology. And, to be sure, the apparatus does provide renewed hope for people with diabetes. Still, the "hybrid" qualifier is an important one, especially when weighing biogenetic factors against informatic necessities. The machine still requires consistent input from users who need to enter mealtime carbohydrates (as they would typical insulin injections), accept bolus recommendations to correct high blood sugars, and (in most cases) calibrate the sensor on at least a daily basis, which requires using a glucometer. Despite all its advantages, the closed-loop system demands a more activated patient, not one prone to apathy and neglect. Medtronic created a website for the device to engage consumer questions and it was immediately inundated by prospective buyers. The first inquiry came from a person who hoped the device would decrease the number of finger pricks needed on any given day. If the system is a "closed loop," then surely the sensor would accurately gauge blood sugars. But when a company representative responded that she did not know how frequently the user tested their blood sugars, another forum member noted that Medtronic's own materials declared, "All therapy adjustments should be based on measurements obtained using a home blood glucose monitor and not on values provided by the Guardian Sensor." In other words, ever more finger pricks. Another asked, "But if the incorporated CGM is used to drive the insulin pump and you cannot be certain of the BG gauge, how safe is the entire system?" Within a month the site had received accolades from consumers eager to adopt the technology as well as concerns from others about the effectiveness of the device. Inquiries were often mundane, addressing everything from the tubing mechanisms employed to the weight of the machine to the water resistance of the device. One interlocutor remarked that the sensors for the CGM did not stay in place while exercising. Another person complained that insurance did not cover enough of the cost being demanded by the company. And yet another observed that approximating carbohydrates is an inevitably flawed practice, especially if one frequents restaurants. A final participant eschewed the technology entirely because he did not want to use any device that required two infusion sites. He said bluntly, "I do not want to be a walking cyborg."

Perhaps most depressing was the shaming and reiterating of disciplinary scripts that haunted the forum. Even in a space dedicated to moving discussions of diabetes forward, the locus on personal responsibility and projections of excessiveness and guilt persisted. A poster named Wendy scolded a person with type 2 diabetes who wanted to know why the device would not be more widely prescribed. Wendy retorted: "I didn't cause Type 1 Diabetes. I didn't ask for it. No warning was given to my parents that they would need to give injections to their baby girl. In fact no amount of exercise or healthy eating will ever change what is the truth. And that truth is my pancreas doesn't work . . . This is the difference as to why this wouldn't work for you as a Type 2 Diabetic. Lifestyle changes are essential for Type 2 Diabetics." The comments are perplexing not only because plenty of people with type 2 diabetes use insulin pumps but also because there is no shortage of materials to construct the machines. The politics of scarcity and the desire for moral purity and segmentation apart from people who bring shame upon themselves surfaces even in situations where it is decidedly out of place. As I have noted throughout this book, falsehoods that suggest type 2 is easily managed and type 1 is inherently calamitous persisted. Even with the most cutting-edge technology available, there are reliable traces of tropes that situate people as lazy and obtuse, figures that have been with us for decades. The unease associated with type 1diabetes also materialized when respondents expressed worry about DKA and the potentially fatal nature of the device. The despondency of having to constantly enact performances of the agentic subject, even when attached to a machine, was reflected by a user named Trent who argued the science was evolving too slowly. Trent lamented, "So it's basically a CGM and an insulin pump. The only adjustment is that they communicate? This took decades to figure out?" Lest we think the hybridity of the body is moving at an accelerated pace, some people long to be more fully integrated as cyborg. Here the machines finally share communion as the human awaits transformation.

If the artificial pancreas seems like a space-aged dream come to life, it already feels like a relic compared to futuristic devices being cultivated to aid in management efforts. In one recent development, researchers with GoogleX, the team that invented Google Glass, are exploring the possibilities of using a contact lens–like device that would measure glucose through a person's tears.[58] The apparatus would employ a microscopic wireless chip and a miniaturized glucose sensor, which would be embedded between two layers of soft contact lens material. The chip and sensor would be akin to "flakes of glitter," exacerbating the blurred line between the physical and non-physical realms of being in miniaturized fashion.[59] An antenna thinner than a human hair would connect to an external pump to calculate the needed amount of glucose or insulin. The lens would perform a reading every second and be equipped with a safety mechanism to ensure balanced amounts of both substances. And while Google does not have the systematized networks of expertise employed by large pharmaceutical companies, analysts also note that the tech conglomerate is not known for augmenting technology halfheartedly.[60] Google has also been pioneering a bandage-like device that is worn on the skin to monitor glucose using a CGM. As with the contact lens, the appliance would alleviate the need for people with diabetes to perform finger pricks. Perhaps most noteworthy in this venture is that Google will facilitate a "cloud-based system" that will store glucose readings, making the information available for users at any time and at any place.[61] Important questions remain about where that information will be stored, who will have access to it, and how it might be used.

The joining of machine and person, of physical and non-physical elements alike, points to a future that is both fantastical and humbling. The connections among informatics, biologics, and capitalism continue to grow stronger, even as diabetes remains an incurable and frequently unmanageable disease. Although technology provides an important glance into the future, we should not forget that Haraway was also concerned with the mediation of political action—hoping the figure of the cyborg would provide opportunities for openness and possibilities worth embracing. Those affinity politics are not always readily discernable in rhetorics about diabetes and technology, certainly not in the same ways they were identifiable to feminist politics decades ago. Nonetheless, such political alternatives are vital and I address them in the final section of this chapter. Activists must make interventions into the market or there will be few people who can afford the innovations being produced. At the top of that list is the extraordinarily high cost of insulin.

Bittersweet: Consumerism, Advocacy, and the Future of Diabetes Management

In the final months of 2016 there was a sharp uptick in the number of news stories decrying the high cost of insulin. The once affordable medication climbed 300 percent in less than a decade, a daunting increase for countless people who depend on it to survive. The corporate greed that has catalyzed insulin's high cost is a glaring regulatory failure of the American healthcare system, being criticized by advocacy groups, medical practitioners, and members of Congress alike.[62] Once characterized by biblical allusions such as the "Lazarus" effect, insulin has quickly become a metaphor for corporate debasement and the unending appetite for profiting from the misfortunes of others. In the introduction to this book I noted that diabetes is often personified by hazardous figures such as stalkers and terrorists. This comparison has quickly moved to pharmaceutical companies themselves, with one mother telling NBC news, "I feel like they're holding my kid ransom."[63] And indeed they are. Insulin is as vital as water and air and placing it out of reach is tantamount to a hostage situation that will play out in due time. Unfortunately, the US government does not negotiate with terrorists. As a result, people living with diabetes are often left to their own devices while the stewards of capitalism play Russian roulette with their health. It is not enough to hope that multinational corporations will suddenly adopt charitable dispositions. The high cost of being ill requires institutional interference, aggressive regulatory policies, and changes in cultural attitudes about care. In addition, the divides among people with types 1 and 2 diabetes must be resisted, as a sustained focus on government action is required to contain profit-driven exploitation. Although such evolutions would no doubt unfold slowly, there are signs that indicate the ways we approach diabetes are changing and those reconfigurations can muster the rhetorical resources for thinking politics anew.

Creating systemic change demands a multipronged approach to diabetes management, including those steps that rest on the institutional level and those that emanate from below. Of course, a focus on something like vernacular language strategies to supplant egregious capitalist enterprises can feel like an exercise in academic charades when addressing major problems with the healthcare system. But if we are to move beyond the "activated patient" and "passive consumer" dualism that tends to haunt medical literature, then attention must be paid to those places where transformative possibilities lurk.[64] This book outlined four heuristics for contemplating diabetes management, and this chapter has revisited three of them: fantasies of unconscious control, the fatalism of disease, and the always desired agentic subject. Less emphasis has been given to the communal interests served by attending to chronic disease. The tendency to ground diabetes management in a language stressing individualism has a strong gravitational pull, and contemplating productive strategies for centering the body politic remains a challenge. Further emphasis on community investments in health care can and should propagate rhetorics that extol investments in institutions, such as the ones exhibited in the previous chapter, and perform significant political and cultural work when attending to public health. Investing in diabetes care means making resources available to those struggling with the disease, rendering advocacy organizations more visible, and forcing the government to be responsive to the multi-headed beast that constitutes diabetes. To be sure, this agenda may seem as utopian as the technologies discussed in this chapter. Donald Trump's presidency continues to imperil the Affordable Care Act, a landmark piece of legislation that has provided health care to tens of millions of people, which could be gutted with the stroke of a pen. The recent debates over the high cost of insulin provide one flashpoint for thinking through the benefits of more stringent regulatory oversights and point to a lexicon that can facilitate incremental changes in culture.

The sheer rate at which insulin prices have skyrocketed is staggering. Dr. Mayer Davidson, a professor of medicine who studies the insulin market, told one news source that the cost of insulin "borders on the unbelievable." He observed that in 2001 the wholesale price of a month's supply of insulin was roughly $45. In 2016 that same supply cost patients about $1,447.[65] This rapid escalation stems in part from the fact that only three corporations produce insulin: Eli Lilly, Novo Nordisk, and Sanofi. These manufacturers have steadily raised the cost of insulin simultaneously, making claims that competition lowers prices dubious.

In fact, between the third quarters of 2008 and 2016, the price of insulin was raised sixteen times, and ten of those increases happened at the same moment and for the exact same amount.[66] The companies tend to blame high insurance deductibles for medical expenses but generally have little to say about the price gouging in which many diabetes organizations implicate them. Although insurance helps many people pay for insulin, it rarely covers the entire bill. People who lose their jobs or who do not qualify for public assistance are often forced to resort to desperate measures, such as charging hundreds of dollars on credit cards, to pay for medicine.[67] In the face of such exploitation, corporate public relations hacks resort to self-congratulatory platitudes, such as a spokesperson for Eli Lilly who contended the company prices insulin "based on the value" it brings "to patients, providers, payers, and society."[68] The invocation of society seems especially suspicious when we consider the altruistic roots that brought insulin to the market. Three of the men credited with discovering insulin sold their shares of the patent for one dollar each so that the medicine could be mass-produced and made widely available. Of course, the "value" described by Lilly's representative is not a consequence of a "natural" supply and demand fever dream, but a consistently manipulated market to inflate earnings. And, to no one's surprise, all three of the pharmaceutical companies continue to report astounding profits. At the heart of that profiteering is a process known as "evergreening."

If insulin was once heralded for its mythic scientific ethos, literally lifting people from the grave, this resurrection trope today is pertinent for an entirely different reason: the revitalization and extension of patents through the practice of "evergreening." In this manufacturing tactic, corporations incrementally alter the composition of a medication and proclaim it an original innovation to market a product anew. There is nothing inherently illegal about the technique, though the ethics of evergreening continues to receive scrutiny from watchdog groups and critics of the pharmaceutical industry. Still, evergreening rarely brings benefits to patients. It exists so that manufacturers can maintain market shares and mitigate the effects of generics on their bottom lines. It has proven to be an effective strategy. Studies find that 90 percent of privately insured people with type 2 diabetes are prescribed the newest and most expensive products, a direct result of evergreening's consequences.[69] To be fair, some scholars have rightfully pointed out that many of insulin's evolutionary turns were significant enough to not fit squarely in the accusatory frame that accompanies "evergreening."[70] But there have been few recent innovations in insulin science, and sales of the substance continue to yield billions in profits annually.[71] Slight changes to patent formulas have permitted an unchecked spree of consumer fleecing.[72] Even more surprising, as Green and Riggs argue, is that older insulin products have never emerged as competitive generics. Instead, those insulins were rendered obsolete and "promptly removed from the US market."[73]

The slow death that denotes life with diabetes is eerily parallel to the gradual escalation of insulin prices in the United States. As costs rise, patients are often pressured to dial down the amount of insulin they take to ensure their supplies stretch from month to month. Evergreening has confounded these problems by prohibiting the creation of a generic insulin, despite that fact that it was discovered more than a century ago. Nearly 80 percent of all prescriptions written in the United States are generics, indicating a demand for off-brand insulin. The lack of choice and control of the market by a few conglomerates places people with diabetes in the position of always looking to the next great innovation, lest they, like the boy in the Humulin advertisement, remain living in the past. Although some older variants of insulin are available for a cheaper cost, they do not always make for an easy way of life. So long as government regulatory agencies continue to ignore evergreening and the restraints it puts on research to create "biosimilars," the technical name for "generic" insulin, many people with diabetes will continue making trade-offs: medicine or mortgage, health care or hunger?[74] These are the stakes when diabetes care is not systemically addressed.

Despite all of these problems, I believe there are rhetorical resources for engaging the everyday realities of diabetes management. The advent of a term such as evergreening, for example, reveals a capitalist innovation that, once named, can be critiqued and resisted. Just as Haraway suggested that her manifesto was not programmatic but sought to generate "all kinds of linguistic possibilities for politics" that were rarely considered, subtle shifts in meaning can serve pragmatic ends. Evergreening presents a starting point for consumer watch groups and diabetes organizations that wish to highlight practices that consistently wreak havoc on communities, not simply individuals. Even the ACA has provided a springboard for contemplating policies that were not widely circulated before it came into existence. Terms like "single payer" and "universal health care," for example, rarely made appearances in popular media outlets engaging community commitments to care but have become fixtures of news reports and political talk shows. The normalizing of such language provides hope, however small, for the years to come. Likewise, giving presence to problematic frames such as the agentic subject and the ease of diabetes management offers productive starting points for thinking through vernacular responses to the disease.

The pushback on corporations that place the cost of insulin out of reach is already evident in a variety of settings. The American Diabetes Association is lobbying Congress to address the burdensome cost of insulin, and the JDRF continues to fight for innovations such as the artificial pancreas. Forumites to the new Medtronic device were quick to argue that the corporation owed its customers a debt of gratitude for the billions it has made from them. One poster argued that the cutting-edge technology "should be free to the thousands of people that have paid you millions, possibly billions of dollars over the years. How can a company like yours sleep at night knowing this? That is all! PS: 38 year T1 Diabetic (I knew what pork and beef insulin injections were!)." Another user contended the "entire industry revolves around money and this is just the next step to make extra dollars with fancy new devices that don't do anything miraculously different." Of course, I have no illusions that Medtronic is going to turn over tens of thousands of devices at no cost to people with diabetes. I turn to this rhetoric for signs that resistance is possible and not outside the scope of collective action. The history of diabetes management provides a blueprint for thinking the world otherwise, sometimes by reminding us how profits are privileged over people. The resistance to typical approaches to diabetes can be found in the efforts of the community blog Beyond Type 1, the work of the International Diabetes Federation (IDF), and organizations such as Insulin for Life USA. The IDF notes that 415 million adults have diabetes, that between 80,000 and 100,000 children with diabetes do not have access to medicine, and that a person with diabetes dies every six seconds somewhere in the world. The necessity to act is more pressing than ever.

The cyborg sensibilities outlined in this chapter evince both radical retorts to the gallows of capitalism but also the necessity of making due with the daily complexities of a condition like diabetes. The cost of insulin, CGMs, insulin pumps, and other technologies will continue to remain out of reach for scores of people until residents demand government regulations on the pharmaceutical industry or until state actors take the initiative to place regulatory checks on the multinational corporations that make these commodities. I'm not optimistic that either of these will happen imminently. The recent debate over the ACA offers a cautionary tale. Despite the popularity of the ACA, few citizens are single-issue voters on matters of health care. Even with appeals to protect those with pre-existing conditions, which captures a universality not reserved for specific illnesses or disabilities, the particularity of diseases like diabetes will continue being relegated to the trappings of individuated management regimens. And, of course, those with private healthcare insurance are not always quick to check the worst impulses of capitalism run amok. Whether citizens fear losing insurance privileges, believe another person is taking what they feel is rightfully theirs, or are simply overwhelmed by the mammoth task of fighting the stewards of capitalism, the potential for transformative systemic action feels distant, even if possibilities for resistance remain.

Without political intervention, I expect a preponderance of despairing figurations about diabetes to proliferate. The tendency to invoke apocalyptic rhetoric, underscored by precariously positioned bodies, will continue unabated. Statistics that relay the slow death of populations, sometimes articulated to racialized or economically marginalized people, will be reproduced in an unrelenting fashion. The biopolitical tendency to live and let live, in order to ensure that pharmaceutical companies reap profits, will endure. Lest we think all is lost, organizations such as the JDRF illustrate that the trope of fatalism can be appropriated to infiltrate cultural fantasies of agentic actors with complete control over their bodies and their environments. Still, we are a long way from replacing a lexicon of management that emphasizes restraint and personal transcendence. The need to scrutinize representations of diabetes is an ongoing project that requires scholarly flexibility, both in approach and method. As this study has shown, it is easy to arrive at conclusions about diabetes and the people who live with it when those assessments are not rendered in situ. Looking to the ways meaning-making practices enact specific figurations of diabetes accentuates the tropological tripping that Haraway celebrated and brings us closer, little by little, to addressing the confounding nature of the disease. Giving presence to struggles over meaning-making is vital to attending to the opportunities and constraints provided by diabetes rhetoric, as such practices have unending implications for the ways people understand policy choices, medical vernacular, and the moral worth of people. Mining the productive possibilities of discourses across contexts can muster the critical vocabulary for scrutinizing diabetes's many forms. A metaphor such as "epidemic" can be deterministically fatalistic, yes, but it can also function to marshal invaluable resources. Individual success managing diabetes can prop up fictional notions of individualism, but also demarcate systemic failures. Moving forward, people with diabetes must continue circulating their experiences with the disease to ensure the multifaceted nature of the condition is contemplated as a product of culture, not simply biology or genetics. Change comes gradually, but transformations to diabetes management can happen, and have. The parlance of diabetes management is a composite structure, not a monolith, and for some their greatest resources for instigating change lie in their experiences. If only someone listens.

ACKNOWLEDGMENTS

I hate having diabetes. I recognize there are more polite ways to communicate that sentiment, but probably none that are as forthright or sincere. I hate the constant monitoring of my body. I hate the bouts of severe hypoglycemia in the middle of the night. I hate how those sleepless nights make me feel the next day. I hate navigating airport security while wearing technologies that are meant to keep me alive. I hate the shots, and the finger pricks, and the blood draws, and the carb counting, and the cost of prescriptions, and the judgments made by other people. I especially hate the judgment. I hate diabetes so much that it actually startles me that I managed to write a book about it. This task was accomplished, no doubt, because of the amazing community of people who have provided encouragement, support, and kind words as this project has developed. Both writing and living with a chronic illness can be lonely endeavors, and I've benefited from the friendship and confidence of a good many people. I hate having diabetes but, because of the wonderous care offered by those around me, I really enjoyed the process of thinking about its materialization in everyday life.

To start, many of the ideas I explore in this book were initially delivered to Communication Studies departments who graciously invited me to discuss the concept of diabetes management. I want to thank the community of scholars at Indiana University, the University of Illinois, the University of Wisconsin, Northwestern University, and the University of Pittsburgh for offering the time and space for contemplating this work with me and making it decidedly stronger in the process.

I also want to thank Vanderbilt University and the University of Iowa for providing research leaves that gave me the time to read, write, and think about the themes in this book. The Communication Studies departments at both Vanderbilt and Iowa have amazing communities of scholars, and I am grateful for the generosity and love they have shown to both me and my work. At Vanderbilt I have the pleasure of keeping the company of Vanessa Beasley, Neil Butt, Stephanie Covington, Bonnie Dow, Bohyeong Kim, Claire King, John Koch, ML Sandoz, John Sloop, Paul Stob, Courtney Travers, Isaac West, and Dustin Wood.

Portions of chapter 4 were originally published in the *Quarterly Journal of Speech*, and parts of chapter 5 were published in the *Journal of Medical Humanities*. I thank the publishers of those journals for allowing my scholarship to be reproduced here.

I am especially appreciative of Ilene Kalish at NYU Press for her keen editorial guidance throughout this process. And thanks also to Jen Jacobs for allowing me to reprint her paintings in the introductory chapter.

Countless people have moved this project to completion by discussing with me the theory incorporated in the book, its case studies, and its implications for broader cultural critique. They are too numerous to name here, which is itself an indication of how lucky I am to have the job that I do. Still, to name just a few: in the subdiscipline of the rhetoric of health and medicine, this project has benefited from the feedback of Lora Arduser, T. Kenny Fountain, Scott Graham, Jennell Johnson, John Lynch, and J. Blake Scott. I am also fortunate to call an amazing group of scholars my academic kin and I am especially thankful to those who have repeatedly engaged the ideas in this book. They include Caitlin Bruce, Cara Buckley, E Cram, Natalie Fixmer-Oraiz, Michaela Frischherz, David Hingstman, Bob Ivie, Brook Irving, Paul Johnson, Jiyeon Kang, John Lucaites, Rachel McLaren, David Moscowitz, Chuck Morris, Jeff Motter, Phaedra Pezzullo, Jamie Skerski, Darrel Wanzer-Serrano, Sue Stanfield, Ted Striphas, Robert Terrill, and Phil Voight. Ann Westerlund, Ryan Petersen, and Matt King provided hours of needed distraction in Nashville. A special thanks to Suzanne Enck and Claire King who, more than any others, have listened to my ideas, read my work, and made me smile constantly throughout this journey.

My family continues to be an amazing source of energy and strength. My parents, siblings, in-laws, and nieces and nephews are nothing short of fabulous. The kids sometimes ask me to test my blood sugar in front of them, and I appreciate being a source of entertainment and not abject horror.

Finally, this book is dedicated to Isaac West because it simply would not have been without him. On the days I hated this project, he stressed how important he thought it was. On the days I was unsure about ideas, he talked through them with me. And on the days I was apprehensive about the methods, or the examples, or the archive, he reminded me that I would not write a text unless it was just a little bit queer. I say again what I said a decade ago: My world is made brighter by his love, his encouragement, and, most especially, his laughter.

NOTES

CHAPTER 1. CRITICAL CONDITIONS

1. Though "illness" is sometimes defined as a subjective measurement of human experience and "disease" a more objective component of the medical model, chronic conditions such as diabetes trouble such easy classifications.
2. A "normal" reading for blood sugar in people without diabetes is usually signified by the number 90.
3. Annemarie Mol, *The Logic of Care: Health and the Problem of Patient Choice* (New York: Routledge, 2008), 54.
4. For two excellent personal narratives that engage a multitude of variables, see Sonia Sotomayor, *My Beloved World* (New York: Vintage, 2014) and Tim Anderson, *Sweet Tooth: A Memoir* (Seattle, WA: Lake Union, 2014).
5. See also Helene Shugart, *Heavy: The Obesity Crisis in Cultural Context* (New York: Oxford University Press, 2016).
6. See Richard Klein, "What Is Health and How Do You Get It?," in *Against Health: How Health Became the New Morality* (New York: New York University Press, 2010), 15–25.
7. Paula Treichler, *How to Have Theory in an Epidemic: Cultural Chronicles of AIDS* (Durham, NC: Duke University Press, 1999).
8. There is an immense body of work on all of these topics and little room to expand on each of them here. Some examples include, Christophe M. Filippi and Matthias G. von Herrath, "Viral Trigger for Type 1 Diabetes: Pros and Cons," *Diabetes* 57 (2008): 2863–2871; Giovanni Musso, Roberto Gambino, and Maurizio Cassader, "Obesity, Diabetes, and Gut Microbiota: The Hygiene Hypothesis Expanded?," *Diabetes Care* 33 (2010): 2277–2284; Veronica G. Parker, Rachel M. Mayo, Barbara N. Logan, Barbara J. Holder, and Patricia T. Smart, "Toxins and Diabetes Mellitus: An Environmental Connection?," *Diabetes Spectrum* 15 (2002): 109–112.
9. Etymologically condensation simply means "the act of making more dense." Condensation is used in fields such as rhetorical studies to describe the compression of multiple referents, attitudes, or expressions into a singular form. This "composite structure" is often affective in its execution and used as a standard for judgment. See John Story, *Cultural Theory and Popular Culture: An Introduction* (New York: Routledge, 2006), 73.
10. Phaedra Pezzullo points out that breast cancer activism often adopts perspectives that are conservative and progressive simultaneously and that to truly understand

breast cancer's actualization in the public sphere we must examine both sides of that coin. See "Resisting 'National Breast Cancer Awareness Month': The Rhetoric of Counterpublics and their Cultural Performances," *Quarterly Journal of Speech* 89 (2003): 347.

11 National Center for Chronic Disease Prevention and Health Promotion, "National Diabetes Statistics Report," June 10, 2014, http://www.cdc.gov.
12 Patrick Lustman, "Depression in Adults with Diabetes," *Psychiatric Times*, January 1, 2002.
13 American Diabetes Association, "Economic Cost of Diabetes in the U.S. in 2017," *Diabetes Care*, March 22, 2018, http://care.diabetesjournals.org.
14 Kelly Close, "Diabetes, A Silent Threat to US Economy," *TheHill.com*, April 7, 2015, http://thehill.com; Susan Blumenthal, "Obesity: America's Next Great National Security Threat?," *Huffington Post*, June 8, 2012, http://www.huffingtonpost.com.
15 The "Four-H" groups were Haitians, hemophiliacs, homosexuals, and heroin users.
16 Some medical practitioners have begun to use the term "late adult-onset" to distinguish from the more common term "juvenile diabetes." As one sign that management rhetorics still reflect such biases, when I was initially diagnosed months before turning thirty, I was given a Pink Panther coloring book to instruct me about the ramifications of diabetes.
17 See "Signs of Diabetes in Children," JDRF, http://www.jdrf.org.
18 Kevin Ferguson, "The Cinema of Control: On Diabetic Excess and Illness in Film," *Journal of Medical Humanities* 31 (2010): 183–204.
19 To be more specific, at first the pancreas may over-produce insulin to make up for the insulin resistance the body is experiencing.
20 David Kendall, "With Diabetes, Don't Focus on Blame," *CNN.com*, April 15, 2011.
21 American Diabetes Association, "Diabetes Myths," http://www.diabetes.org. See also Gina Kolata, "Obesity May Be Only One Piece of Diabetes Puzzle," *New York Times*, August 20, 2007.
22 The genealogy of "management" is traceable to disparate traditions preoccupied with the regulation of the self and the controlling of the passions. Inflect the term management with "restraint," for example, and it can be easily linked to the Greek Stoics with their emphasis on consciously sober judgments to best navigate the world. Restraint might beckon inquiries by sociologists such as Norbert Elias, who studied the gradual conditioning of the self in social situations, always leaving room for individual agency in networked structures. It could bring to bear Freud's notions of the superego and resisting impulses of the id. Contemporary notions of management might also be attached to relics of scientific investigation, such as those avowed by thinkers like Frederick Taylor, in which the scientific method was applied to labor to increase productivity and revolutionize work practices, but with less than satisfying results for workers. Due to space constraints, I do not engage all of these traditions, but each is arguably significant to the study of management's parameters.

23 Robert Steinbrook, "Facing the Diabetes Epidemic—Mandatory Reporting of Glycosylated Hemoglobin Values in New York City," *New England Journal of Medicine* 354 (2006): 546.
24 Melissa Hunter and Dana King, "COPD: Management of Acute Exacerbations and Chronic Stable Disease," *American Family Physician* 64 (2001): 603–613.
25 P. G. Kopelman and C. Grace, "New Thoughts on Managing Obesity," *Gut: A Journal of Gastroenterology and Hepatology* 53 (2004): 1044–1053.
26 Although there is little space here to detail how each of these is put into discourse, all of them are couched in management terms in diffuse places. The CDC makes reference to managing epilepsy, coronary artery disease, diabetes, obesity, and asthma, among others.
27 See, for example, Thomas Frieden, Moupali Das-Douglas, Scott Kellerman, and Kelly Henning, "Applying Public Health Principles to the HIV Epidemic," *New England Journal of Medicine* 353 (2005): 2397–2402; Cathryn Domrose, "Changing Face of AIDS," *Nurse Week*, September 6, 2001.
28 David Morris, *Illness and Culture in the Postmodern Age* (Berkeley: University of California Press, 1998).
29 Zoltan Majdik and Carrie Ann Platt, "Selling Certainty: Genetic Complexity and Moral Urgency in Myriad Genetics' BRAC Analysis Campaign," *Rhetoric Society Quarterly* 42 (2012): 131.
30 Alan Petersen and Deborah Lupton, *The New Public Health: Discourse, Knowledges, Strategies* (London: SAGE, 1996), 61.
31 Arthur Kleinman, *The Illness Narratives: Suffering, Healing, and the Human Condition* (New York: Basic Books, 1989).
32 Peter Conrad, *The Medicalization of Society* (Baltimore, MD: Johns Hopkins University Press, 2007), 8.
33 Mary Specker Stone, "In Search of Patient Agency in the Rhetoric of Diabetes Care," *Technical Communication Quarterly* 6 (Spring 1997): 202.
34 Stone, "In Search of Patient Agency," 208.
35 Steve Ferzacca, "'Actually, I Don't Feel That Bad: Managing Diabetes and the Clinical Encounter," *Medical Anthropology Quarterly* 14 (2000): 28–50.
36 Mol, *Logic of Care*, 43.
37 Amy Borovoy and Janet Hine, "Managing the Unmanageable: Elderly Russian Jewish Émigrés and the Biomedical Culture of Diabetes Care," *Medical Anthropology Quarterly* 22 (2008): 3.
38 The idea of vernacular rhetoric is often understood as a form of localized knowledge that is contrasted to popularly circulated knowledge or discourse employed by powerful figures. I use it here more colloquially to refer to cultural norms that reinforce and are reinforced by knowledge that is often partial, filtered through a lens of "common sense," and adopted from a variety of sources.
39 See Lora Arduser, *Living Chronic: Agency and Expertise in the Rhetoric of Diabetes* (Columbus: Ohio State University Press, 2017), 165.

40. Annemarie Mol and John Law, "Embodied Action, Enacted Bodies: The Example of Hypoglycemia," *Body and Society* 10 (2004): 50.
41. Morris, *Illness and Culture in the Postmodern Age*, 6.
42. Arthur Frank and Therese Jones, "Bioethics and the Later Foucault," *Journal of Medical Humanities* 24 (2003): 179.
43. Borovoy and Hine, "Managing the Unmanageable," 10
44. Lennard J. Davis, *Enforcing Normality: Disability, Deafness, and the Body* (New York: Verso, 1995), 130.
45. Thomas Insel, "No Health Without Mental Health," National Institute of Mental Health, September 6, 2011, https://www.nimh.nih.gov.
46. Mol, *Logic of Care*, 19.
47. Petersen and Lupton, *The New Public Health*, 72.
48. For more on breast cancer awareness campaigns see Pezzullo, "Resisting National Breast Cancer Awareness Month"; Lisa Keränen, *Scientific Character: Rhetoric, Politics, and Trust in Breast Cancer Research* (Tuscaloosa: University of Alabama Press, 2010); Kelly E. Happe, *The Material Gene: Gender, Race, and Heredity After the Human Genome Project* (New York: New York University Press, 2013); Samantha King, *Pink Ribbons Inc.: Breast Cancer and the Politics of Philanthropy* (Minneapolis: University of Minnesota Press, 2006).
49. Peter Conrad and Rochelle Kern, *Sociology of Heath and Illness: Critical Perspectives* (New York: Worth, 2005), 4.
50. This is especially true for people who lack access to health insurance. Lydia Ramsey, "Diabetics Can Spend $1,000 a Month Taking Care of Themselves—And It's Not Just Because of Insulin," *Businessinsider.com*, September 19, 2016, http://www.businessinsider.com.
51. Anahad O'Connor, "Economic Toll of Diabetes Begins Early," *New York Times*, January 9, 2012.
52. Janet Jakobsen, "Queer Is? Queer Does? Normativity and the Problem of Resistance," *GLQ* 4 (1998): 519.
53. Anselm Strauss, "America: In Sickness and Health," *Society* 10 (1973): 33. Strauss goes on to define chronic conditions as "slow-acting, long term killers that can be treated but not cured." He is keen to note that chronic conditions are products of everyday communication and not pure medical knowledge. As a result, chronic conditions are not always easy to delimit.
54. Conrad, *The Medicalization of Society*, 152.
55. Jakobsen, "Queer Is? Queer Does?," 518.
56. Emily Martin, "The Egg and the Sperm: How Science Has Constructed a Romance Based on Stereotypical Male-Female Roles," *Signs: Journal of Women in Culture and Society* 16 (1991): 485–501.
57. I am following the lead of scholars such as Ann Cvetkovich in situating management as a key word. See her book *Depression: A Public Feeling* (Durham, NC: Duke University Press, 2012); for Raymond Williams's most explicit treatment of a "structure of feeling," see *Marxism and Literature* (New York: Oxford University Press, 1977).

58 Beth Howard, "More Pre-Med Students Opting for Health Humanities Programs," *Association of American Medical Colleges News*, December 12, 2016, https://news.aamc.org.
59 Belinda Jack, "The Rise of Medical Humanities," *Times Higher Education*, January 22, 2015.
60 Sarah Atkinson, Bethan Evans, Angela Woods, and Robin Kearns, "'The Medical' and 'Health' in a Critical Medical Humanities," *Journal of Medical Humanities* 36 (2015): 71–72.
61 Keränen, *Scientific Characters*, 23.
62 John Lynch, *What Are Stem Cells?: Definitions at the Intersection of Science and Politics* (Tuscaloosa: University of Alabama Press, 2011), 5.
63 For a notable exception, see Alan Graber, Anne W. Brown, and Kathleen Wolff, *A Life of Control: Stories of Living with Diabetes* (Nashville, TN: Vanderbilt University Press, 2010).
64 Martha Cooper and Carole Blair, "Foucault's Ethics," *Qualitative Inquiry* 8 (2002): 513.
65 Lauren Berlant and Michael Warner, "Sex in Public," *Critical Inquiry* 24 (1998): 547–566.
66 For more on "absent archives," see Cvetkovich, *Depression*.
67 For more on the intersection of queer theory and crip theory, see Robert McRuer, *Crip Theory: Cultural Signs of Queerness and Disability* (New York: New York University Press, 2006); James L. Cherney and Kurt Lindemann, "Queering Street: Homosociality, Masculinity, and Disability in Friday Night Lights," *Western Journal of Communication* 78 (2014): 1–21.
68 One exemplar is Petra Kuppers's study of Shimon Attie's *White Nights, Sugar Dreams*, an art installation whose object is diabetes, which provides one possibility for critically engaging the public character of the disease. The installation is set in a dark room with three monitors. Visitors hear multiple narratives of people with diabetes being interviewed, but never see their faces. Instead, patrons watch videos of evolving landscapes on a screen, which features a red liquid that changes shape as white crystals fall into it. The red and white represent blood and sugar respectively, and Kuppers observes how the faux glucose fluidly climbs into mountainous shapes, providing new perspectives on diabetes. For Kuppers, the aural narratives and the visual promiscuity of the sugar reveal new ways of gauging what is happening on the inside of the body, but not privileging typical medical epistemologies. The installation centralizes the lives of those with diabetes. The narratives themselves craft a multiplicity of experiences, giving attention to a community creation where "no one way of living with diabetes puts itself at center stage." The interactive nature of the installation ensures that the piece is experiential, where "the movement of everyday life can work against the fixing stare or the observing gaze historically associated with modern medicine." Art can replot public receptions of disease and illness, instigating novel perspectives through incongruous posturing or proffering a vernacular that fundamentally alters our

equipment for living. *The Scar of Visibility: Medical Performances and Contemporary Art* (Minneapolis: University of Minnesota Press, 2007), 47–53.
69   Mol, *Logic of Care*, 77.
70   Lauren Berlant, *The Queen of America Goes to Washington City: Essays on Sex and Citizenship* (Durham, NC: Duke University Press, 1997), 12.

CHAPTER 2. "HIV IS THE NEW DIABETES"
 1   Daniel Villarreal, "Is Having HIV Really Just Like Having Diabetes or Being Short?," *Queerty*, September 9, 2011, http://www.queerty.com.
 2   Richard Klein reminds us that the rhetorical parameters of health are decidedly more difficult to define than the contours of illness. See "What Is Health and How Do You Get It?," in *Against Health: How Health Became the New Morality*, ed. Jonathan Metzl and Anna Kirkland (New York: New York University Press, 2010), 15–25.
 3   Berlant, "Slow Death (Sovereignty, Obesity, Lateral Agency)," *Critical Inquiry* 33 (2007): 759.
 4   Debates over pre-exposure prophylaxis (PrEP), a technology that has proven to be highly effective in preventing HIV transmission, is just one area where the paranoia underlying comparisons to diabetes is especially strong.
 5   Chaïm Perelman, *The Realm of Rhetoric* (South Bend, IN: University of Notre Dame Press, 1990).
 6   Isaac West, "Analogizing Interracial and Same-Sex Marriage," *Philosophy and Rhetoric* 48 (2015): 561–582.
 7   For an elongated history of diabetes see Chris Feudtner, *Bittersweet: Diabetes, Insulin, and the Transformation of Illness* (Chapel Hill: University of North Carolina Press, 2003).
 8   Jean Scandlyn, "When AIDS Became a Chronic Disease," *Western Journal of Medicine* 172 (2000): 130–133.
 9   Paula Treichler, *How to Have Theory in an Epidemic: Cultural Chronicles of AIDS* (Durham, NC: Duke University Press, 1999); Susan Sontag, *Illness as Metaphor and AIDS and Its Metaphors* (New York: Picador, 1989), 104–112. Sontag looks specifically to syphilis and cancer when discussing analogies to HIV/AIDS.
10   Eve Kosofsky Sedgwick, *Touching Feeling: Affect, Pedagogy, Performativities* (Durham, NC: Duke University Press, 2003); Cvetkovich, *Depression*.
11   Robert McRuer and Anna Mollow, *Sex and Disability* (Durham, NC: Duke University Press, 2012); McRuer, *Crip Theory*.
12   Ellis Hanson, "The Future's Eve: Reparative Reading After Sedgwick," *South Atlantic Quarterly* 110 (2011): 113.
13   I have noted elsewhere the enduring history that conjoins AIDS, apocalyptic rhetoric, and the ambivalent effects this sensibility has on LGBT movement trajectories. See Jeffrey A. Bennett, "Queer Teenagers and the Mediation of Utopian Catastrophe," *Critical Studies in Media Communication* 27 (2010): 455–476.
14   Thomas Long, *AIDS and American Apocalypse: Cultural Semiotics of an Epidemic* (Albany: State University of New York Press, 2005), 18.

15 Peter Dickinson, "Go-go Dancing on the Brink of the Apocalypse," in *Postmodern Apocalypse: Theory and Cultural Practice at the End*, ed. R. Dellamora (Philadelphia: University of Pennsylvania Press, 1995), 219.
16 For some examples of this trope see Long, *AIDS and American Apocalypse*; David Savran, "Tony Kushner Considers the Longstanding Problems of Virtue and Happiness," *American Theatre* 11 (1994): 20–27, 100–104.
17 Barry Brummett, *Contemporary Apocalyptic Rhetoric* (New York: Praeger, 1991), 91.
18 Although characteristically imagined with regard to religious groups, fragments of apocalypse surface in diffuse aspects of American social movements. This is significant, Robyn Wiegman tells us, because Left politics had been infiltrated by the nostalgia of 1960s identity movements that consistently positioned themselves as having lost the "utopian generation of a future tense." See "Feminism's Apocalyptic Futures," *New Literary History* 31 (2000): 805–807.
19 Brummett, *Contemporary Apocalyptic Rhetoric*, 86.
20 Wiegman, "Feminism's Apocalyptic Failures," 807.
21 The FDA's current policy requires that all men who have sex with men are to refrain from donating blood if they have had sex with another man in the past year.
22 C. Riley Snorton, *Nobody Is Supposed to Know: Black Sexuality on the Down Low* (Minneapolis: University of Minnesota Press, 2014).
23 Eve Kosofsky Sedgwick, "Paranoid Reading and Reparative Reading, or, You're So Paranoid, You Probably Think This Essay Is About You," in *Touching Feeling: Affect, Pedagogy, Performativity* (Durham, NC: Duke University Press, 2003).
24 Sedgwick noted, "I daily encounter graduate students who are dab hands at unveiling the hidden historical violences that underlie a secular, universalist liberal humanism. Yet these students' sentient years, unlike the formative years of their teachers, have been spent entirely in a xenophobic Reagan-Bush-Clinton-Bush America where "liberal" is, if anything, a taboo category and where "secular humanism" is routinely treated as a marginal religious sect, while a vast majority of the population claims to engage in direct intercourse with multiple invisible entities such as angels, Satan, and God." In *Touching/Feeling*, 139–140.
25 Sedgwick, "Paranoid and Reparative Reading," 149.
26 Such impulses are also found in celebratory queer scholarship. For example, in a special issue of *Criticism* dedicated to Sedgwick's memory, Heather Love reflects on the unconscious reverberations effecting her scholarly tendencies. "In my case, I am hailed as one of the latecomers to queer theory who picks up paranoid habits of mind as critical tools or weapons but is detached from the living contexts in which these frameworks were articulated (primarily, the AIDS crisis of the 1980s)." Likewise, Hanson points to Gary Fisher, a gay black man who died of AIDS and whose biography troubles many queer scholars who see nothing but paranoid possibilities in his supposedly contemptible desires and sexual practices. See Love, "Truth and Consequences: On Paranoid Reading and Reparative Reading," *Criticism* 52 (2010): 236.

27 Randy Martin, "A Precarious Dance, a Derivative Sociality," *TDR: The Drama Review* 56 (2012): 62.
28 Judith Butler, "Performativity, Precarity, and Sexual Politics," *AIBR: Revista de Antropología Iberoamericana* 4 (2009): ii.
29 Berlant, "Slow Death."
30 See, for example, Lauren Berlant and Lee Edelman, *Sex, or the Unbearable* (Durham, NC: Duke University Press, 2014), 35–61.
31 Butler, "Performativity, Precarity, and Sexual Politics," xiii.
32 Berlant, "Slow Death."
33 Jasbir Puar, ed., "Precarity Talk: A Virtual Roundtable with Lauren Berlant, Judith Butler, Bojana Cvejić, Isabell Lorey, Jasbir Puar, Ana Vujanović," *TDR: The Drama Review* 56 (2012): 163–177.
34 *Nip/Tuck*, television series. "Willy Ward," season 4, episode 14. Directed by Michael Robin. Original air date December 5, 2006.
35 James Gavin, "Barebacking: Baring the Truth," *Out*, July 25, 2007; Sebaspace, "Bareback Porn Is Back!" *Afrogay.blogspot.com*, February 10, 2011.
36 Quoted in Virgil Dickson, "AIDS Funding Cuts Stirring Fears," *Herald News*, August 5, 2008.
37 John Ryan, "Increased Risk for Type-2 Diabetes Mellitus with HIV-1 Infection," *Insulin* 5 (2010): 37–45.
38 Bonnie Dow, "Criticism and Authority in the Artistic Mode," *Western Journal of Communication* 65 (2001): 340.
39 Dennis Rhodes, "Taking Care," *The Body*, March 1999.
40 AIDS Policy and Law, "What If HIV Becomes a Manageable Condition?" 14 (1999): 11.
41 Clint Walters, "Disclosing HIV?," *PositiveNation* 135 (2007).
42 Margie Mason, "San Francisco AIDS Activists Angry at Disease's Evolution," *Desert News*, June 3, 2001.
43 Paige Parker, "Guessing About HIV May Keep Epidemic Going," *The Oregonian*, October 13, 2007.
44 Andrew Sullivan, "Still Here, So Sorry," *The Advocate*, July 5, 2005, 72.
45 Andrew Sullivan, "Why Aren't Gay Men on the Pill?," *The Dish*, April 9, 2014.
46 Andy Oehler, "Letter to the Editor," *The Advocate*, August 16, 2005, 22.
47 Thomas Gegeny, "Letter to the Editor," *The Advocate*, August 16, 2005, 22.
48 Joe Perez, "How to Prevent AIDS: My Response to Andrew Sullivan," *Soulfully Gay, Part Two*, May 23, 2005.
49 Michael Fein, "Letter to the Editor," *The Advocate*, August 16, 2005, 22.
50 John-Manuel Andriote, "HIV Is 'Like Diabetes'? Let's Stop Kidding Ourselves," *Huffington Post*, January 1, 2012.
51 See Walters, "Disclosing HIV?."
52 Berlant, "Slow Death," 776.
53 Julian Weitzenfeld, "Valid Reasoning by Analogy," *Philosophy of Science* 51 (1984): 137–149.

54 S. Scott Graham, *The Politics of Pain Medicine: A Rhetorical-Ontological Inquiry* (Chicago: University of Chicago Press, 2015), 129.
55 See Chris Hayes, "All In," *MSNBC*, June 13, 2016; Tom Dyer, "Positive Message: Bob Poe Wants to Put a Positive Face on HIV in Congress," June 9, 2016, http://www.watermarkonline.com; Dan Avery, "Congressional Candidate Bob Poe Comes Out as HIV-Positive," *NewNextNow*, June 11, 2016, http://www.newnownext.com.
56 See Dyer, "Positive Message."
57 See "Congressional Candidate Bob Poe Says He's HIV Positive," June 10, 2016, http://sandrarose.com.
58 Max Pemberton, "As a Doctor I'd Rather Have HIV than Diabetes," *The Spectator*, April 19, 2014.
59 Likewise, Dr. Joe Wright reflected on the words of a cardiologist who contended, "Even so, I'd choose to have HIV over diabetes." The physician has rationalized that a regimen to eradicate diabetes remains more difficult than the management of HIV. He argues that HIV can be regulated by taking a pill, inverting the above equation.
60 Sedgwick, "Paranoid and Reparative Reading," 149.
61 For more on the debates about shame in LGBTQ circles, see Erin Rand, *Reclaiming Queer: Activist and Academic Rhetorics of Resistance* (Tuscaloosa: University of Alabama Press, 2014): 127–155.
62 Clay Wirestone, "What People with Type-One Diabetes can Learn from Type 2s," *DiabetesHealth.com*, April 19, 2010.
63 Julie Deardorff, "Diabetes' Civil War: People with Type 1 Diabetes, Outnumbered and Overshadowed by Type 2, Fight for Recognition, Resources—and a New Name for Their Disorder," *Chicago Tribune*, November 22, 2010, http://articles.chicagotribune.com.
64 River Solomon, "I Have Diabetes. Am I to Blame?," *New York Times*, October 12, 2016, http://www.nytimes.com.
65 Cvetkovich, *Depression*.
66 Mark Smith, "The AIDS Dilemma," *Liberty Report*, May 1987, 3.
67 Michael Chapman, "AFA: Gay Sex 'Is Dangerous to Your Health'—Why Won't Obama Advise Gays to Stop It to Avoid AIDS?," *csnnews.com*, June 23, 2016, http://www.cnsnews.com.
68 Chris Beyrer, "The Global Response to HIV in Men Who Have Sex with Men," *Lancet* 388 (2016): 198–206; Free and Equal: United Nations for LGBT Equality, "Fact Sheet: Criminalization," https://www.unfe.org.
69 Breanne Fahs, "Daddy's Little Girls: On the Perils of Chastity Clubs, Purity Balls, and Ritualized Abstinence," *Frontiers: A Journal of Women Studies* 31 (2010): 116–142.
70 Diabetes is not the only phenomenon that might be read as simultaneously still and contagious. David Cisneros has captured how media often frame immigrants similarly. See "Contaminated Communities: The Metaphor of 'Immigrant as

Pollutant' in Media Representations of Immigration," *Rhetoric and Public Affairs* 11 (2008): 569–602.
71 Gene Demby, "Who's Really Left Out of the CrossFit Circle," *National Public Radio*, September 13, 2013, http://www.npr.org.
72 Alexander Wolf and Nancy Liu, "The Numbers of Shame and Blame: How Stigma Affects Patients and Diabetes Management," *diaTribe*, August 7, 2014, http://diatribe.org.
73 Sontag, *Illness as Metaphor*, 113.
74 Kathleen LeBesco, *Revolting Bodies? The Struggle to Redefine Fat Identity* (Amherst: University of Massachusetts Press, 2004), 87.
75 To be sure, blanket racial classifications can be as problematic as erasures, omitting significant information about social class and economic well-being. Arleen Marcia Tuchman has persuasively argued that factors such as socioeconomic class continue to be disregarded in the collecting of data about diabetes rates, and such omissions mask the lethal nature of diabetes more generally. See Tuchman, "Diabetes and Race: A Historical Perspective," *American Journal of Public Health* 101 (2001): 24–33.
76 Andrew Sullivan, "When Plagues End," *New York Times Magazine*, November 10, 1996.
77 See Phillip Brian Harper, *Private Affairs: Critical Ventures in the Culture of Social Relations* (New York: New York University Press, 1999); C. Riley Snorton, *Nobody Is Supposed to Know*; Cathy Cohen, *The Boundaries of Blackness: AIDS and the Breakdown of Black Politics* (Chicago: University of Chicago Press, 1999).
78 Snorton, *Nobody Is Supposed to Know*, 12.
79 Kevin Mumford, *Not Straight, Not White: Black Gay Men from the March on Washington to the AIDS Crisis* (Chapel Hill: University of North Carolina Press, 2016).
80 Cathy Cohen, "Black Sexuality, Indigenous Moral Panics, and Respectability: From Bill Cosby to the Down Low," in *Moral Panics, Sex Panics*, ed. Gilbert Herdt (New York: New York University Press, 2009), 113.
81 Mark Polite, "Bill Cosby's 'Tough Love' is Counterproductive," *Time.com*, June 12, 2013, http://ideas.time.com.
82 The source of type 1 diabetes is mysterious at best and scientifically opaque at worst. Most authorities believe the catalyst for disease is a combination of both genetics and the environment, though the exact relationship among them is unknown, as are the environmental triggers. The American Diabetes Association reports that, "In most cases of type 1 diabetes, people need to inherit risk factors from both parents." Researchers, however, also acknowledge that most people who are at risk for diabetes never develop it, leading them to look for an environmental impetus that brings type 1 diabetes into being. The most frequently employed explanation is that an intruder, such as a virus, incites the immune system. Alongside viruses, some experts propose cold weather might instigate diabetes because the disease develops most often in the winter months and is more preva-

lent in cooler climates. It could also be that diet early in life is a contributing factor. Scientists have found that type 1 diabetes is "less common in people who were breastfed and in those who first ate solid foods at later ages." More recently, it has been speculated that a degree of bodily trauma, at any point in life, might "flip the switch" on the disease. As these examples illustrate, the stationary view of diabetes can be countered even prior to the materialization of disease. Contingency is far from conceptual here, being a central and mysterious agent in the condition's emergence.

83 Troy Duster, *Backdoor to Eugenics* (New York: Routledge, 2003); Kelly E. Happe, *The Material Gene: Gender, Race, and Heredity After the Human Genome Project* (New York: New York University Press, 2013).
84 Sontag, *Illness and Metaphor*; Treichler, *How to Have Theory in an Epidemic*.
85 Michael Hanne and S. J. Hawken, "Metaphors for Illness in Contemporary Media," *Medical Humanities* 33 (2007): 93–99.
86 Jordan Lite, "City Stalked by Diabetes," *NYDailyNews.com*, July 25, 2007, http://www.nydailynews.com.
87 Kas Thomas, "Alzheimer's Is Type-Three Diabetes," *bigthink.com*, September 10, 2014.

CHAPTER 3. LETHAL PREMONITIONS

1 The JDRF is known only by its acronym to reflect the fact that most people with type 1 diabetes are not children.
2 Allen Spiegel, "The Stem Cell Wars: A Dispatch from the Front," *Transactions of the American Clinical and Climatological Association* 124 (2013): 94–110, http://www.ncbi.nlm.nih.gov.
3 Offering presence to the fatalism that underwrites the JDRF's rhetoric is not meant to suggest that the hearings are punctuated in their entirety by despair. Rather, the organization's rhetoric cannot be understood devoid of considerations of fatalism.
4 The 2007 hearings do not have a video archive.
5 See Eve Kosofsky Sedgwick, "How to Bring Your Kids Up Gay," *Tendencies* (Durham, NC: Duke University Press, 1993): 154–164; Kathryn Boyd Stockton, *The Queer Child: Or Growing Sideways in the Twentieth Century* (Durham, NC: Duke University Press, 2009); Judith Halberstam, *The Queer Art of Failure* (Durham, NC: Duke University Press, 2011); Lee Edelman, *No Future: Queer Theory and the Death Drive* (Durham, NC: Duke University Press, 2004).
6 Jeffrey A. Bennett, "Queer Teenagers and the Mediation of Utopian Catastrophe," *Critical Studies in Media Communication* 27 (2010): 455–476.
7 Stockton, *The Queer Child*, 16.
8 Charles E. Morris III, "Sunder the Children: Abraham Lincoln's Queer Rhetorical Pedagogy," *Quarterly Journal of Speech* 99 (2014): 395–422.
9 Brian Amsden, "Negotiating Liberalism and Bio-Politics: Stylizing Power in Defense of the Mall Curfew," *Quarterly Journal of Speech* 94 (2008): 407–429.

10 danah boyd, *It's Complicated: The Social Lives of Networked Teens* (New Haven, CT: Yale University Press, 2014).
11 Chris Feudtner, *Bittersweet: Diabetes, Insulin, and the Transformation of Illness* (Chapel Hill: University of North Carolina Press, 2003), 6–10.
12 Lauren Berlant, *The Queen of America Goes to Washington City: Essays on Sex and Citizenship* (Durham, NC: Duke University Press, 1997), 223.
13 Michel Foucault, *Fearless Speech* (Los Angeles: Semiotext(e), 2001).
14 In the first session, spending was voted down 37–63; in the second 42–57; in the third 48–52. US Congress, Senate, Committee on Appropriations, *Juvenile Diabetes: Hearing Before the Subcommittee on Labor, Health and Human Services, and Education, and Related Agencies* [hereinafter *Juvenile Diabetes*], 106th Congress, 1999, 2 (statement of Sen. Arlen Specter).
15 US Congress, Senate, Committee on Homeland Security and Governmental Affairs, *Juvenile Diabetes: Examining the Personal Toll on Families, Financial Costs to the Federal Health Care System, and Research Progress Toward a Cure* [hereinafter *Examining the Personal Toll 2005*], 109th Congress, 2005, 11 (statement of Mary Tyler Moore, International Chair, JDRF).
16 *Juvenile Diabetes*, 3 (statement of Sen. Larry Craig).
17 *Examining the Personal Toll 2005*, 27 (statement of Sen. Susan Collins).
18 *Examining the Personal Toll 2005*, 28 (statement of Sen. Frank Lautenberg).
19 *Examining the Personal Toll 2005*, 28–29 (statement of Sen. Frank Lautenberg).
20 Dhruv Khullar, "The Trouble with Medicine's Metaphors," *The Atlantic*, August 7, 2014, http://www.theatlantic.com.
21 US Congress, Senate, Permanent Subcommittee on the Investigations of the Committee on Governmental Affairs, *Diabetes: Is Sufficient Funding Being Allocated to Fight This Disease?* [hereinafter *Is Sufficient Funding Being Allocated*], 107th Congress, 2001, 4 (statement of Sen. Carl Levin).
22 *Is Sufficient Funding Being Allocated*, 5 (statement of Sen. Jean Carnahan).
23 US Congress, Senate, Committee on Governmental Affairs, *Juvenile Diabetes: Examining the Personal Toll on Families, Financial Costs to the Federal Health Care System, and Research Progress Toward a Cure: Hearing Before Governmental Affairs* [hereinafter *Examining the Personal Toll 2003*], 108th Congress, 2003, 6 (statement of Sen. Robert Bennett).
24 In 1999, Senators Mack and Specter tied diabetes back to personal experiences with cancer. *Juvenile Diabetes*, 17 (statement of Sen. Connie Mack); *Juvenile Diabetes*, 17–18 (statement of Sen. Arlen Specter).
25 The JDRF fosters relationships with members of Congress by inviting them and their families to act as co-chairs to the Children's Congress. For example, Rep. Tom Osborne (NE) was the chair-dad of the Children's Congress in 2003. Sen. Jeanne Shaheen's daughter Stephanie and son-in-law Craig were co-chairs in 2011.
26 US Congress, Senate, Committee on Homeland Security and Governmental Affairs, *Transforming Lives Through Diabetes Research* [hereinafter *Transforming Lives*], 112th Congress, 2011, 3–4 (statement of Sen. Susan Collins).

27 *Juvenile Diabetes*, 25 (statement of Sen. Harry Reid); *Examining the Personal Toll 2005*, 7 (statement of Sen. Frank Lautenberg).
28 Each hearing has unique features despite the sometimes-repetitive form. The celebrities that testify, concurrent events on Capitol Hill, and the political conditions inspiring the lobbying efforts all give each event a specific flavor. The 1999 hearings found politicians coming and going from the room because of espionage hearings. Another year the Senate was impeaching a federal judge at the same time JDRF members were testifying.
29 *Juvenile Diabetes*, 19 (statement of Mary Tyler Moore). The official government transcript has Moore saying "30,000" children will be diagnosed with diabetes each year. However, another statistic frequently invoked at these hearings is thirty-five children diagnosed daily. Thirty-five each day for a year would be about 12,775 children, which is just under 13,000, which sounds like 30,000. It is likely that the transcript is incorrect. The JDRF reports that Moore simply confused her statistics.
30 She did it at every hearing from 2003 to 2011.
31 *Is Sufficient Funding Being Allocated*, 5 (statement of Sen. Daniel Akaka); 12 (statement of James Lovell); 17 (statement of Allen Spiegel, director, National Institute of Diabetes and Digestive and Kidney Diseases, National Institutes of Health).
32 US Congress, Senate, Committee on Homeland Security and Governmental Affairs, *The Juvenile Diabetes Research Foundation and the Federal Government: A Model Public-Private Partnership Accelerating Research Toward a Cure* [hereinafter *JDRF and the Federal Government*], 110th Congress, 2007, 13 (statement of Adam Morrison); 20 (statement of Caroline McEnery); 24 (statement of Ann Strader).
33 US Congress, Senate, Committee on Homeland Security and Governmental Affairs, *Type 1 Diabetes Research: Real Progress and Real Hope for a Cure* [hereinafter *Type 1 Diabetes Research*], 111th Congress, 2009, 16 (statement of Nicholas Jonas); 23 (statement of Ellen Gould).
34 *Transforming Lives*, 29 (statement of Kerry Morgan).
35 *Examining the Personal Toll 2005*, 9 (statement of Mary Tyler Moore).
36 *Type 1 Diabetes Research*, 24 (statement of Ellen Gould).
37 *Is Sufficient Funding Being Allocated*, 7 (statement of Mary Tyler Moore).
38 *Is Sufficient Funding Being Allocated*, 7 (statement of Mary Tyler Moore).
39 The metaphor of the time bomb would be employed by Moore again in 2003 and 2005. *Examining the Personal Toll 2003*, 10; *Examining the Personal Toll 2005*, 11.
40 *Juvenile Diabetes*, 19 (statement of Mary Tyler Moore).
41 *Examining the Personal Toll 2003*, 7 (statement of Mary Tyler Moore).
42 *Examining the Personal Toll 2003*, 8 (statement of Mary Tyler Moore).
43 *Examining the Personal Toll 2003*, 8 (statement of Mary Tyler Moore).
44 *Type 1 Diabetes Research*, 22 (statement of Asa Kelly). Emphasis mine.

45 *Examining the Personal Toll 2005*, 24 (statement of Aaron Jones). Emphasis mine.
46 *JDRF and the Federal Government*, 19 (statement of Caroline McEnery).
47 *Juvenile Diabetes*, 31 (statement of Will Smith).
48 *JDRF and the Federal Government*, 22 (statement of Tré Hawkins).
49 *Examining the Personal Toll 2003*, 19 (statement of Sophia Cygnarowicz).
50 *Juvenile Diabetes*, 28 (statement of Stockton Morris).
51 *Juvenile Diabetes*, 30 (statement of Molly Singer).
52 *Is Sufficient Funding Being Allocated*, 28 (statement of Rachel Dudley).
53 *Examining the Personal Toll 2003*, 22 (statement of LaNiece Evans-Scott).
54 *Is Sufficient Funding Being Allocated*, 33 (statement of Caroline Rowley).
55 *Is Sufficient Funding Being Allocated*, 33–34 (statement of Caroline Rowley).
56 *Examining the Personal Toll 2003*, 23 (statement of Eric Bonness).
57 *Examining the Personal Toll 2003*, 24 (statement of Colleen Rea, on behalf of her son Dylan Rea).
58 *JDRF and the Federal Government*, 21 (statement of Caitlin Crawford).
59 *Is Sufficient Funding Being Allocated*, 30 (statement of Andrew Webber).
60 *Examining the Personal Toll 2003*, 17 (statement of Katie Halasz).
61 *Is Sufficient Funding Being Allocated*, 22 (statement of LaNiece Evans-Scott).
62 See Michel Foucault, *The History of Sexuality, Vol. 1: An Introduction*. Translated by Robert Hurley (New York: Vintage Books, 1990), 146.
63 *Juvenile Diabetes*, 30 (statement of Molly Singer).
64 *Examining the Personal Toll 2003*, 19 (statement of Sophia Cygnarowicz).
65 *Examining the Personal Toll 2005*, 26 (statement of Lauren Stanford).
66 As will be explored in the conclusion, insulin pumps offer a mechanism for control, but are no guarantee without the participation of a highly motivated and vigilant patient.
67 *Juvenile Diabetes*, 10–11 (statement of Harold Varmus, director of the National Institute of Health).
68 John Lynch, *What Are Stem Cells?: Definitions at the Intersection of Science and Politics* (Tuscaloosa: University of Alabama Press, 2011), 124.
69 *Is Sufficient Funding Being Allocated*, 23 (statement of Sen. Susan Collins).
70 Scientists have long hoped that stem cells could be engineered to develop into islet-like cells that would produce insulin. That research is ongoing.
71 *Examining the Personal Toll 2005*, 3 (statement of Sen. Susan Collins).
72 *Is Sufficient Funding Being Allocated*, 19 (statement of Hugh Auchincloss, Jr., Professor of Surgery, Massachusetts General Hospital and Harvard Medical School).
73 *Examining the Personal Toll 2005*, 2 (statement of Sen. Susan Collins).
74 Most islet transplant recipients require insulin again after two years. See David M. Harlan, "Islet Transplantation for Hypoglycemia Unawareness/Severe Hypoglycemia: Caveat Emptor," *Diabetes Care* 39 (2016): 1072–1074. Thanks to Dr. Allen Spiegel for directing me to this citation.
75 *Is Sufficient Funding Being Allocated*, 17 (statement of Allen Spiegel).

76 *Examining the Personal Toll 2003*, 31 (statement of Bernhard Hering, Associate Professor of Surgery, Director of Islet Transplantation, University of Minnesota).
77 *Examining the Personal Toll 2003*, 31 (statement of Bernhard Hering).
78 *Examining the Personal Toll 2005*, 10 (statement of Mary Tyler Moore).
79 *Examining the Personal Toll 2005*, 11 (statement of Mary Tyler Moore).
80 Not only did the stonewalling of resources inhibit a cure for diabetes, it set a precedent for determining which grants the government would fund. Researchers worried the policy would have detrimental effects on a generation of scientists who often select their field of study based on their ability to obtain a first grant. Since most scientists receive their first major grant from the government, the freeze was thought to have a chilling effect on the career decisions of young scientists. Not to be outdone, the JDRF put into place a successful training program for pediatric endocrinologists, providing career development to those who studied type 1 diabetes in children. See Auchincloss, *Is Sufficient Funding Being Allocated*, 24 (statement of Hugh Auchincloss).
81 *Examining the Personal Toll 2005*, 13 (statement of Douglas Wick, film producer and co-head, Red Wagon Entertainment).
82 *Is Sufficient Funding Being Allocated*, 20 (statement of Hugh Auchincloss).
83 *Juvenile Diabetes*, 14 (statement of Harold Varmus).
84 *JDRF and the Federal Government*, 14 (statement of Griffin Rodgers, director, National Institute of Diabetes and Digestive and Kidney Diseases, NIH).
85 *Transforming Lives*, 13 (statement of Charles Zimliki, chairman, Artificial Pancreas Critical Path Initiative, Center for Devices and Radiological Health, Food and Drug Administration).
86 Perhaps one of the most compelling aspects of Zimliki's testimony is the frequency with which industry comes up. Industry is rarely foregrounded in these conversations and its presence here is unusual. *Transforming Lives*, 14 (statement of Charles Zimliki).
87 *Transforming Lives*, 13 (statement of Charles Zimliki).
88 *Transforming Lives*, 14 (statement of Charles Zimliki).
89 *Transforming Lives*, 27 (statement of Caroline Jacobs).
90 *Transforming Lives*, 25 (statement of Sen. Mark Begich).
91 Of course, both Medtronic and the state of Massachusetts stand to make millions from an expedited process.
92 *Transforming Lives*, 18 (statement of Sen. Scott Brown).
93 Zimliki, *Transforming Lives*, 20 (statement of Charles Zimliki).
94 *Transforming Lives*, 20 (statement of Sen. Jeanne Shaheen).
95 *Transforming Lives*, 29 (statement of Kerry Morgan).
96 *JDRF and the Federal Government*, 20 (statement of Caroline McEnery).
97 *JDRF and the Federal Government*, 20 (statement of Caroline McEnery).
98 *Transforming Lives*, 25 (statement of Sen. Mark Begich).
99 *Type 1 Diabetes Research*, 26 (statement of Patrick Gould).

100 US Congress, Senate, Special Committee on Aging, *Diabetes Research: Reducing the Burden of Diabetes at All Ages and Stages* [hereinafter *Diabetes Research*], 113th Congress, 2013 (statement of Sen. Ben Nelson).
101 *Diabetes Research* (statement of Sen Ben Nelson).
102 *Diabetes Research* (statement of Sen. Ben Nelson).
103 *Diabetes Research* (statement of Ray Allen).

CHAPTER 4. CONTAINING SOTOMAYOR

1 Jeffrey Rosen, "The Case Against Sotomayor," *New Republic*, May 4, 2009, https://newrepublic.com; John Derbyshire, "Essentialist Jurisprudence," *National Review Online*, May 4, 2009, https://www.nationalreview.com.
2 The most famous version of the speech was given at a 2001 memorial lecture for the University of California, Berkeley, School of Law. See Sonia Sotomayor, "A Latina Judge's Voice," *Berkeley La Raza Law Journal* 13 (2002): 87–93, http://scholarship.law.berkeley.edu.
3 Peter Baker and Jeff Zeleny, "Obama Chooses Hispanic Judge for Supreme Court Seat," *New York Times*, May 26, 2009, http://www.nytimes.com.
4 See Rosen, "The Case Against Sotomayor"; Derbyshire, "Essentialist Jurisprudence."
5 Karen Tumulty, "Sonia Sotomayor and Type-One Diabetes," *Time*, May 27, 2009, http://swampland.time.com.
6 As the National Institute of Diabetes and Digestive and Kidney Diseases (NIDDK) points out, "People will have different A1C targets depending on their diabetes history and their general health." See "The A1C Test and Diabetes," September 2014, https://www.niddk.nih.gov.
7 Linda Martín Alcoff, "Sotomayor's Reasoning," *Southern Journal of Philosophy* 48 (2010): 122–138; José Esteban Muñoz, "Wise Latinas," *Criticism* 56 (2014): 249–265.
8 Lisa Flores, "Between Abundance and Marginalization: The Imperative of Racial Rhetorical Criticism," *Review of Communication* 16 (2016): 13.
9 Josue David Cisneros, *The Border Crossed Us: Rhetorics of Borders, Citizenship, and Latina/o Identity* (Tuscaloosa: University of Alabama Press, 2014), 146.
10 W.J.T. Mitchell, "Seeing Disability," *Public Culture* 13 (2001): 395.
11 On diabetes and personal agency, see Lora Arduser, *Living Chronic: Agency and Expertise in the Rhetoric of Diabetes* (Columbus: Ohio State University Press, 2017).
12 Amy Borovoy and Janet Hine, "Managing the Unmanageable: Elderly Russian Jewish Émigrés and the Biomedical Culture of Diabetes Care," *Medical Anthropology Quarterly* 22 (2008): 10.
13 Lisa Duggan, in "Proliferating Cripistemologies: A Virtual Roundtable," ed. Robert McRuer and Merri Lisa Johnson, *Journal of Literary and Cultural Disability Studies* 8 (2014): 166.
14 See Cassandra Jackson, "Visualizing Slavery: Photography and the Disabled Subject in the Art of Carrie Mae Weems," in *Blackness and Disability: Critical*

Examinations and Cultural Interventions, ed. Chris Bell (East Lansing: Michigan State University Press, 2011), 31–46; Sharon Snyder and David T. Mitchell, *Cultural Locations of Disability* (Chicago: University of Chicago Press, 2006); Ellen Samuels, *Fantasies of Identification: Disability, Gender, Race* (New York: New York University Press, 2014).

15 See Chris Bell, "Doing Representation Work," in *Blackness and Disability: Critical Examinations and Cultural Interventions*, ed. Chris Bell (East Lansing: Michigan State University Press, 2011): 1–2.

16 Subini Ancy Annamma, David Connor, and Beth Ferri, "Dis/Ability Critical Race Studies (DisCrit): Theorizing at the Intersection of Race and Dis/ability, *Race Ethnicity and Education* 16 (2013): 1–31; "Proliferating Cripistemologies: A Virtual Roundtable," ed. Robert McRuer and Merri Lisa Johnson, *Journal of Literary and Cultural Disability Studies* 8 (2014): 149–169.

17 Chávez and Griffin, "Introduction: Standing at the Intersection of Feminisms, Intersectionality, and Communication Studies," in *Standing in the Intersection: Feminist Voices, Feminist Practices in Communication Studies*, ed. Karma Chávez and Cindy Griffin (Albany: State University of New York Press, 2012), 2.

18 Chávez and Griffin, "Introduction," 8.

19 Sara McKinnon, "Essentialism, Intersectionality and Recognition: A Feminist Rhetorical Approach to the Audience," in Chávez and Griffin, *Standing in the Intersection*, 190.

20 McKinnon, "Essentialism, Intersectionality, and Recognition," 192.

21 Bonnie Dow, "Authority, Invention, and Context in Feminist Rhetorical Criticism," *Review of Communication* 16 (2016): 60–76.

22 Dow, "Authority, Invention, and Context in Feminist Rhetorical Criticism," 66.

23 Leslie Hahner, "Constitutive Intersectionality and the Affect of Rhetorical Form," in Chávez and Griffin, *Standing in the Intersection*, 155.

24 Hahner, "Constitutive Intersectionality," 147.

25 Troy Duster, *Backdoor to Eugenics* (New York: Routledge, 1990).

26 See Helene Shugart, *Heavy: The Obesity Crisis in Cultural Context* (New York: Oxford University Press, 2016), 80–82; Arleen Marcia Tuchman, "Diabetes and Race: A Historical Perspective," *American Journal of Public Health* 101 (2011): 24–33.

27 Gloria E. Anzaldúa, *Light in the Dark/Luz en lo Oscuro: Rewriting Identity, Spirituality, Reality*, ed. AnaLouise Keating (Durham, NC: Duke University Press Books, 2015); see also Suzanne Bost, *Encarnación: Illness and Body Politics in Chicana Feminist Literature* (New York: Fordham University Press, 2010), 15; AnaLouise Keating, "'Working toward Wholeness': Gloria Anzaldúa's Struggles to Live with Diabetes and Chronic Illness," in *Speaking from the Body: Latinas on Health and Culture*, ed. Angie Chabram-Dernerseian and Adela de la Torre (Tucson: University of Arizona Press, 2008): 133–143.

28 The Sotomayor case may strike some as especially ironic considering the ways the legal system has consistently prohibited appeals based on multiple identity

categories. See Isaac West, *Transforming Citizenships: Transgender Articulations of the Law* (New York: New York University Press, 2014), 110.
29 Carolyn Nielsen, "Wise Latina: Framing Sonia Sotomayor in the General-Market and Latina/o-Oriented Prestige Press," *Howard Journal of Communications* 24 (2013): 124.
30 Rosen, "Case Against Sotomayor."
31 Ta-Nehisi Coates, ""The Meme Builds More," *The Atlantic*, May 6, 2009, http://www.theatlantic.com.
32 Amy Goldstein and Jerry Markon, "Sotomayor Has Said Gender and Ethnicity 'Make a Difference' in Judging," *Washington Post*, May 27, 2009, http://www.washingtonpost.com.
33 Sam Stein, "Sotomayor's Medical History Sparks Wider Debate," *Huffington Post*, May 13, 2009, http://www.huffingtonpost.com.
34 Stein, "Sotomayor's Medical History."
35 David J. Garrow, "Mental Decrepitude on the U.S. Supreme Court: The Historical Case for a 28th Amendment," *University of Chicago Law Review* 67 (2000): 995–1087.
36 Stein, "Sotomayor's Medical History."
37 Stein, "Sotomayor's Medical History."
38 On the articulation of "excess" and racialized bodies, see Kathleen LeBesco, *Revolting Bodies?: The Struggle to Redefine Fat Identity* (Amherst: University of Massachusetts Press, 2004): 54–64; Shugart, *Heavy*, 66–87.
39 Joseph Shapiro, "Diabetes: Is It an Issue for the Supreme Court?," *All Things Considered*, National Public Radio, May 27, 2009, http://www.npr.org.
40 Tom Watkins, "Sotomayor's Diabetes: 'She Overcomes It Every Day,'" CNN.com, May 27, 2009, http://www.cnn.com.
41 Stein, "Sotomayor's Medical History."
42 Denise Grady, "Health Spotlight Is on Diabetes, Its Control and Its Complications," *New York Times*, May 26, 2009, https://www.nytimes.com.
43 Baker and Zeleny, "Obama Chooses Hispanic Judge for Supreme Court Seat."
44 Michael Sauland and Larry McShane, "Like All of Her Life Hurdles, Sonia Sotomayor Shrugs Off Diabetes," *New York Daily News*, May 26, 2009, http://www.nydailynews.com.
45 Michael Powell and Serge Kovaleski, "Sotomayor Rose on Merit Alone, Her Allies Say," *New York Times*, June 4, 2009, https://www.nytimes.com.
46 Sheryl Gay Stolberg, "Court Nominee Manages Diabetes with Discipline," *New York Times*, July 9, 2009, https://www.nytimes.com.
47 Powell and Kovaleski, "Sotomayor Rose on Merit Alone."
48 Stolberg, "Court Nominee Manages Diabetes with Discipline."
49 Goldstein and Markon, "Sotomayor Has Said Gender and Ethnicity 'Make a Difference' in Judging."
50 For more on Latino activism, see Darrel Wanzer-Serrano, *The New York Young Lords and the Struggle for Liberation* (Philadelphia, PA: Temple University Press, 2015).

51 Ellis Cose, "Affirmative Action and Sotomayor's Critics," *Newsweek*, May 29, 2009, http://www.newsweek.com.
52 Benjamin Weiser, "Sotomayor's Recusals Suggest Impartiality," *New York Times*, July 1, 2009, https://www.nytimes.com.
53 Weiser, "Sotomayor's Recusals."
54 Tobin Siebers, *Disability Theory* (Ann Arbor: University of Michigan Press, 2008), 105.
55 Erin C. Tarver, "New Forms of Subjectivity: Theorizing the Relational Self with Foucault and Alcoff," *Hypatia* 26 (2011): 808.
56 On the history of Supreme Court hearings, see Trevor Parry-Giles, *The Character of Justice: Rhetoric, Law, and Politics in the Supreme Court Confirmation Process* (East Lansing: Michigan State University Press, 2006).
57 Udi Sommer, "Representative Appointments: The Effect of Women's Groups in Contentious Supreme Court Confirmations," *Journal of Women, Politics & Policy* 34 (2013): 1–22.
58 See Sylvia Manzano and Joseph D. Ura, "Desperately Seeking Sonia? Latino Heterogeneity and Geographic Variation in Web Searches for Judge Sonia Sotomayor," *Political Communication* 30 (2013): 81–99; Guy-Uriel Charles, Daniel L. Chen, and Mitu Gulati, "Sonia Sotomayor and the Construction of Merit," *Emory Law Journal* 61 (2012): 801–861.
59 US Congress, Senate, Committee on the Judiciary, Confirmation Hearing on the Nomination of Hon. Sonia Sotomayor, to be an Associate Justice of the Supreme Court of the United States [hereinafter *Sotomayor Confirmation*], 111th Congress, 1st Session, 2009, 42 (statement of Sen. Dick Durbin).
60 *Sotomayor Confirmation*, 541 (statement of Theodore Shaw).
61 *Sotomayor Confirmation*, 348 (statement of Sen. Tom Coburn). The official testimony reads, "You will have lots of explaining to do."
62 *Sotomayor Confirmation*, 137 (statement of Sen. Lindsay Graham).
63 *Sotomayor Confirmation*, 120 (statement of Sen. Jon Kyl).
64 *Sotomayor Confirmation*, 13 (statement of Sen. Orrin Hatch); 26 (statement of Sen. Lindsay Graham); 101 (statement of Sen. Jeff Sessions).
65 Tom Goldstein, "Her Justice is Blind," *New York Times*, June 15, 2009.
66 Think Progress, "Right-wing Group Launches TV Ad Claiming Sotomayor Led a Terrorist Organization," July 14, 2009, https://thinkprogress.org.
67 Parry-Giles, *The Character of Justice*, 158.
68 Sumi Cho, Kimberlé Crenshaw, and Leslie McCall, "Toward a Field of Intersectionality Studies: Theory, Applications, and Praxis," *Signs* 38 (2013): 789.
69 *Sotomayor Confirmation*, 388 (statement of Sen. Patrick Leahy).
70 *Sotomayor Confirmation*, 35 (statement of Sen. Sheldon Whitehouse).
71 *Sotomayor Confirmation*, 35 (statement of Sen. Sheldon Whitehouse).
72 Muñoz, "Wise Latinas," 251.
73 *Sotomayor Confirmation*, 142 (statement of Hon. Sonia Sotomayor).
74 *Sotomayor Confirmation*, 377 (statement of Hon. Sonia Sotomayor).

75 *Sotomayor Confirmation*, 359 (statement of Hon. Sonia Sotomayor). Emphasis mine.
76 *Sotomayor Confirmation*, 71 (statement of Hon. Sonia Sotomayor).
77 *Sotomayor Confirmation*, 327 (statement of Hon. Sonia Sotomayor).
78 Terry Maroney, "Angry Judges," *Vanderbilt Law Review* 65 (2012): 1215.
79 Michael Doyle and David Lightman, "What Has Sotomayor Revealed? Self-Control," *St. Paul Pioneer Press*, July 15, 2009, https://www.twincities.com.
80 See the conversation between the *Washington Post*'s Dana Milbank and NPR's Steve Inskeep, "Senators Share Spotlight with Sotomayor," *Morning Edition*, July 15, 2009, https://www.npr.org.
81 Ann Gerhart, "Warming the Room with a Confident Touch," *Washington Post*, July 15, 2009, http://www.washingtonpost.com.
82 Sheryl Gay Stolberg, "Sotomayor Leaves Passion Behind,'" *New York Times*, July 14, 2009, https://www.nytimes.com.
83 Charlie Savage, "A Nominee on Display, but Not Her Views," *New York Times*, July 16, 2009, https://www.nytimes.com.
84 *Philadelphia Inquirer*, "Editorial: A Vote for Sotomayor," July 17, 2009, http://www.philly.com; Michael Goodwin, "Senators, Just Give Sotomayor Her Robe Already," *New York Daily News*, July 14, 2009, http://www.nydailynews.com; Christine M. Flowers, "The Unswoon-worthy Latino," *Philadelphia Daily News*, July 17, 2009, 21.
85 Savage, "A Nominee on Display."
86 Savage, "A Nominee on Display."
87 Sonia Sotomayor, *My Beloved World* (New York: Vintage Books, 2013), 5.
88 Sotomayor, *My Beloved World*, 350.
89 Sotomayor, *My Beloved World*, 98.
90 Sotomayor, *My Beloved World*, 186.
91 Sotomayor, *My Beloved World*, 186.
92 Sotomayor, *My Beloved World*, 222–223.
93 Sotomayor, *My Beloved World*, 319.
94 Sotomayor, *My Beloved World*, 49.
95 Sotomayor, *My Beloved World*, 214.
96 Sotomayor, *My Beloved World*, 285.
97 Sotomayor, *My Beloved World*, 299.
98 Sotomayor, *My Beloved World*, 353.
99 Sotomayor, *My Beloved World*, 126.
100 Sara Sklaroff, "Meeting the Challenges of Diabetes," *Washington Post*, June 2, 2009, http://www.washingtonpost.com.
101 Charles E. Morris III, "Pink Herring and the Fourth Persona: J. Edgar Hoover's Sex Crime Panic," *Quarterly Journal of Speech* 88 (2002): 228–244.
102 Muñoz, "Wise Latinas," 251.
103 Muñoz, "Wise Latinas," 256.
104 Tarver, "New Forms of Subjectivity," 808.

105 New York City Department of Health and Mental Hygiene, "Epi Data Brief," April 2013, https://www1.nyc.gov.

CHAPTER 5. TROUBLED INTERVENTIONS

1. Gordon Mitchell and Kathleen McTigue rightfully point out that the CDC has monitored noninfectious agents, but these outbreaks (gastrointestinal symptoms, melanoma, and mesothelioma) involved environmental causal agents (such as methyomyl, ultraviolet light, and asbestos). "The U.S. Obesity 'Epidemic': Metaphor, Method, or Madness?," *Social Epistemology* 21 (2007): 401–402.
2. Shadi Chamany et al., "Tracking Diabetes: New York City's A1C Registry," *Milbank Quarterly* 87 (2009): 550.
3. Chamany et al., "Tracking Diabetes," 552.
4. Under the New York plan, scores over 9 percent constitute "poorly controlled" blood sugar. Scores under 7 percent are defined as good control.
5. Although the registry continues to operate as a source of research, surveillance, and community planning, the letters have been discontinued as of this writing. Officials at DOHMH communicate that the registry is an ongoing source of vital information, providing data to support innovative approaches to diabetes rates.
6. For more on the relationship between liberalism and civic humanism, see Ronald Beiner, "Citizenship as a Comprehensive Doctrine," *Hedgehog Review* 10 (2008): 23–33; J.G.A. Pocock, "The Ideal of Citizenship Since Classical Times," *Queen's Quarterly* 99 (1992): 35–55.
7. Robert Steinbrook, "Facing the Diabetes Epidemic—Mandatory Reporting of Glycosylated Hemoglobin Values in New York City," *New England Journal of Medicine* 354 (2006): 546.
8. Michel Foucault, *The Birth of the Clinic: An Archaeology of Medical Perception* (New York: Vintage Books, 1973/1994), 25.
9. Susan Sontag, *Illness as Metaphor* (New York: Farrar, Straus and Giroux, 1978); Priscilla Wald, *Contagious: Cultures, Carriers, and the Outbreak Narrative* (Durham, NC: Duke University Press, 2008).
10. This chapter explores texts that engage New York City's DOHMH's diabetes program and that offer structured coherence to the thematic narratives about "the debate" surrounding the registry. This included representative texts from public health journals, publications posted on DOHMH's website, and law journals. Staying close to the emergent themes of "epidemic" and "privacy" from an initial reading of texts, a search of EBSCO and Lexis/Nexis databases was used to uncover additional evidence. To further enhance this study, an interview was conducted with Dr. Shadi Chamany to clarify materials found in the literature.
11. Amy Fairchild, Ronald Bayer, and James Colgrove, editors, *Searching Eyes: Privacy, the State, and Disease Surveillance in America* (Berkeley: University of California Press, 2007), 1.

12 We might also think of this as the "comic frame." Kenneth Burke situates the "comic frame" in opposition to the "tragic frame." The tragic frame is generally couched in a language that sets "dangerous limitations upon our capacity to know." The comic frame, conversely, recognizes the partiality of identifications and desires. In Burke's words, the comic frame enables people "to be observers of themselves, while acting. Its ultimate would not be passiveness, but maximum consciousness." See Kenneth Burke, *Attitudes Toward History* (Berkeley: University of California Press, 1984), 171; Frank Lentricchia, *Criticism and Social Change* (Chicago: University of Chicago Press, 1985), 62.
13 Steinbrook, "Facing the Diabetes Epidemic," 546–547.
14 New York City Department of Public Health and Mental Hygiene, "New Diabetes Report Documents Devastating Effects in New York City," July 24, 2007, http://www.nyc.gov.
15 Mary Ann Banerji and Robyn Stewart, "A Public Health Approach to the Diabetes Epidemic: New York City's Diabetes Registry," *Current Diabetes Reports* 6 (2006): 169.
16 Department of Health and Mental Hygiene, "New Diabetes Report."
17 In 2000, the average length of a diabetes-related hospital stay was 7.9 days, with the average charge of $17,800 per stay. There is a slow but steady trend of declining length of hospital stay and increasing charges per stay. In 1997, the average hospital stay was 8.9 days and the average charge was $15,400. See *New York State Strategic Plan for the Prevention and Control of Diabetes*. Revised March 2008. http://www.health.state.ny.us
18 New York City Department of Public Health and Mental Hygiene, "Diabetes Among New York City Adults," *NYC Vital Signs* 8 (2009): 3. See the report at: http://www.nyc.gov.
19 Harold J. Krent, Nicholas Gingo, Monica Kapp, Rachel Moran, Mary Neal, Meghan Paulas, Puneet Sarna, and Sarah Suma, "Whose Business Is Your Pancreas? Potential Privacy Problems in New York City's Mandatory Diabetes Registry," *Annals of Health Law* 17 (2008): 5.
20 Zachary Bloomgarden, "A1C in New York City," June 12, 2006, http://www.medscape.com/. Notably, poverty alone does not seem to account for the significant rates of diabetes in the city. As one public health scholar put it: "31% of diabetic patients in commercial managed care and 42% in Medicaid Managed Care in New York State have an A1C of greater than 9%, indicative of poor control. Yet only 10% of people with diabetes are aware of their A1C levels." See Amy Fairchild, "Diabetes and Disease Surveillance," *Science* 313 (2006): 175.
21 Shadi Chamany et al., "Telephone Intervention to Improve Diabetes Control: A Randomized Trial in the New York City A1C Registry," *American Journal of Preventative Medicine* 49 (2015): 832–841.
22 Bloomgarden, "A1C."

23 Amy Fairchild and Ava Alkon, "Back to the Future? Diabetes, HIV, and the Boundaries of Public Health," *Journal of Health Politics, Policy, and Law* 32 (2007): 563.
24 Chamany et al., "Tracking Diabetes," 550.
25 The New York program was modeled in part after a successful registry in Vermont, where patients volunteered to participate in the program. According to Fairchild and Alkon, Vermont's registry "evolved from a voluminous and growing literature that suggests that diabetes-management programs can keep the disease markedly more controlled in discrete populations." The program was developed with the help of Nathaniel Clark, a vice president of clinical affairs at the American Diabetes Association. Clark believed the registry would be particularly useful for diabetics who were marginalized from the system and who might benefit from continuous care. The Vermont program has been hailed as a success by many healthcare advocates and provided momentum to the New York plan. Patients in the Vermont program wrote letters of support to officials in New York praising their system and the benefits it brought. Some registries run internally by hospitals also have been met with success. For example, the Intermountain Healthcare in Salt Lake City experimented with an internal diabetes registry and found that over several years the average A1C "decreased from 8.1 percent to 7.3 percent." Others have pointed to the diabetes registry in New Zealand as an example of a successful program, contending that it is credited with decreasing the prevalence of A1C levels over 9 percent "from 34% of patients with diabetes to just 7%." However, it should be noted that nearly 80 percent of New Zealand's healthcare system is funded by the government and is free for qualifying citizens. See Fairchild and Alkon, "Back to the Future," 570; Clarissa G. Barnes, Frederick L. Brancati, and Tiffany L. Gary, "Virtual Mentor: Mandatory Reporting of Noncommunicable Diseases: The Example of the New York City A1c Registry (NYCAR)," *American Medical Association Journal of Ethics* 9 (2007): 829; Banerji and Stewart, "A Public Health Approach to the Diabetes Epidemic," 170.
26 Arthur Frank, "From Sick Role to Narrative Subject: An Analytic Memoir," *Health* 20 (2016): 15.
27 Judy Segal, *Health and the Rhetoric of Medicine* (Carbondale: Southern Illinois University Press, 2005), 19.
28 Segal, *Health and the Rhetoric of Medicine*, 3.
29 Segal borrows heavily from Kenneth Burke, who has famously quipped that "observations" are "but implications of the particular terminology in terms of which the observations are made. In brief, much of what we take as observations about 'reality' may be but the spinning out of possibilities implicit in our particular choice of terms." See Burke, *Language as Symbolic Action* (Berkeley: University of California Press, 1966), 46.
30 Wald, *Contagious*, 3.
31 Wald, *Contagious*, 53.

32. Nancy Tomes, *The Gospel of Germs: Men, Women, and the Microbe in American Life* (Cambridge, MA: Harvard University Press, 1999), 14, 17.
33. Fairchild, Bayer, and Colgrove, "Searching Eyes."
34. Helene A. Shugart, *Heavy: The Obesity Crisis in Cultural Context* (New York: Oxford University Press, 2016).
35. Lisa Keränen, "Addressing the Epidemic of Epidemics: Germs, Security, and a Call for Biocriticism," *Quarterly Journal of Speech* 97 (2011): 224.
36. Chamany et al., "Tracking Diabetes," 547.
37. The Greek root *demos* found in the second half of *epidemic* will no doubt be familiar to those who study rhetorical, philosophical, and political histories.
38. Bloomgarden, "AIC."
39. Barnes, Brancati, and Gary, "Visual Metaphor," 829.
40. Mitchell and McTigue, "The U.S. Obesity 'Epidemic,'" 394.
41. Wald, *Contagious*, 17.
42. Cindy Patton, *Globalizing AIDS* (Minneapolis: University of Minnesota Press, 2002), 39.
43. For many years, public health departments avoided addressing chronic conditions such as diabetes because they did not mimic other disease models. In the instance of cancer, for example, there was a limited mission of looking at incidence and prevalence. See Fairchild and Alkon, "Back to the Future."
44. Chamany et al., "Tracking Diabetes," 566.
45. Banerji and Stewart, "A Public Health Approach to the Diabetes Epidemic," 170.
46. Ali H. Mokdad et al., "The Continuing Epidemics of Obesity and Diabetes in the United States," *Journal of the American Medical Association* 286 (2001): 1195–1200.
47. The emphasis is mine. Michelle Obama, "Michelle on a Mission: How We Can Empower Parents, Schools, and the Community to Battle Childhood Obesity," *Newsweek*, March 2010, http://www.newsweek.com.
48. Sander Gilman, "Representing Heath and Illness: Thoughts for the 21st Century," *Journal of Medical Humanities* 32 (2011): 69–75.
49. Fairchild and Alkon, "Back to the Future," 564.
50. Banerji and Stewart, "A Public Health Approach to the Diabetes Epidemic," 170–171.
51. Patton, *Globalizing AIDS*, 40.
52. Fairchild, Bayer, and Colgrove, *Searching Eyes*, 28.
53. Fairchild, "Diabetes and Disease Surveillance," 176.
54. Fairchild, Bayer, and Colgrove, *Searching Eyes*, 242. Many of the testimonials they borrow from are also used in Wendy Mariner, "Medicine and Public Health: Crossing Legal Boundaries," *Journal of Health Care Law and Policy* 10 (2007): 121–151.
55. Bloomgarden, "A1C."
56. Fairchild and Alkon, "Back to the Future," 571.
57. Janlori Goldman et al., "New York City's Initiative on Diabetes and HIV/AIDS: Implications for Patient Care, Public Health, and Medical Professionalism,"

American Journal of Public Health 98 (2008): 807. See also Thomas Frieden's response: Frieden, "New York City's Diabetes Reporting System Helps Patients and Physicians," *American Journal of Public Health* 98 (2008): 1543.
58 Krent et al., "Whose Business," 14.
59 Margaret Hoppin, "Overtly Intimate Surveillance: Why Emergent Public Health Surveillance Programs Deserve Strict Scrutiny Under the Fourteenth Amendment," *New York Law Review* 87 (2012): 1950–1995.
60 Mariner, "Medicine and Public Health," 122.
61 Fairchild and Alkon, "Back to the Future," 573.
62 Krent et. al., "Whose Business," 18–19.
63 Krent et al., "Whose Business," 19–20.
64 Krent et al., "Whose Business," 31.
65 Hoppin, "Overtly Intimate Surveillance," 1976.
66 To alleviate these concerns, Krent recommended five "safety" implementations: that the statute expressly state that no information contained in the registry may be subject to subpoena (as the city did with HIV and other sexually transmitted infections); that the notification system be based on affirmative consent; that patients be given the right to opt out of future research unless consent is expressively given; that employers and insurance companies be forbidden to inquire about A1C scores; and that physician names not be disclosed.
67 On contract metaphors, see Margaret Somers, *Genealogies of Citizenship: Markets, Statelessness, and the Right to Have Rights* (New York: Cambridge University Press, 2008).
68 Hoppin, "Overtly Intimate Surveillance," 1989.
69 Mariner, "Medicine and Public Health," 122.
70 It is unclear whether the Trump administration and the Republican party will allow this provision of the ACA to remain in place.
71 Krent et al., "Whose Business," 25.
72 Chamany took issue with these arguments, asserting the law and internal DOHMH protocols protected individual information.
73 Hoppin, "Overtly Intimate Surveillance," 1955.
74 Krent notes the federal government has been given broad authority by the Supreme Court to participate in surveillance programs. *Whalen v. Rose* (1977) remains the sole US Supreme Court case that allowed for public health surveillance. See Fairchild, Bayer, and Colgrove, *Searching Eyes*, 27–28.
75 Mariner, "Medicine and Public Health," 147.
76 Mariner, "Medicine and Public Health," 132.
77 Mariner, "Medicine and Public Health," 132.
78 Mariner, "Medicine and Public Health," 148.
79 Rob Stein, "New York City Starts to Monitor Diabetes," *Washingtonpost.com*, January 11, 2006, http://www.washingtonpost.com.
80 Hoppin, "Overtly Intimate Surveillance," 1994.
81 Barnes, Brancati, and Gary, "Virtual Mentor," 829.

82 Fairchild and Alkon, "Back to the Future," 573–574.
83 Goldman, "New York City's Initiative," 808.
84 Goldman, "New York City's Initiative," 809.
85 Goldman, "New York City's Initiative," 809.
86 Chamany et al., "Tracking Diabetes," 559.
87 I want to thank Bruce Gonbeck for his insights on this point.
88 See James C. Scott, *Seeing Like a State: How Certain Schemes to Improve the Human Condition Have Failed* (New Haven, CT: Yale University Press, 1998).
89 Bloomgarden, "A1C."
90 Bloomgarden, "A1C."
91 Jessica Jones, "Beating an Epidemic," *Government Technology*, December 8, 2005, http://www.govtech.com. Found in Fairchild and Alkon, "Back to the Future," 568.
92 Chamany et al., "Tracking Diabetes," 557.
93 Chamany et al., "Tracking Diabetes," 565.
94 Fairchild and Alkon, "Back to the Future," 572
95 Tomes, *Gospel of Germs*, 258.
96 Chamany et al., "Tracking Diabetes," 557.
97 For more on "infantile citizenship" see Lauren Berlant, *The Queen of America Goes to Washington City: Essays on Sex and Citizenship* (Durham, NC: Duke University Press, 1997).
98 Patrick McGeehan, "Blame Photoshop, Not Diabetes, for This Amputation," *New York Times*, January 24, 2012, http://www.nytimes.com.
99 McGeehan, "Blame Photoshop."
100 Victoria Bekiempis, "The Mayor and Health Department Will Keep Scaring You with Gross Obesity Ads," *Village Voice*, February 6, 2012, http://www.villagevoice.com.
101 McGeehan, "Blame Photoshop."

CHAPTER 6. CYBORG DREAMS

1 The bottom of the display acknowledges that the exhibit was produced to recognize the contributions Genentech has made to the Smithsonian.
2 "Human" insulin generally refers to insulin created in a laboratory. "Human analogue" insulin is also manufactured artificially but genetically engineered to allow for different rates of absorption by users.
3 For more on the relationship between frontier rhetoric and scientific progress, see Leah Ceccarelli, *On the Frontier of Science: An American Rhetoric of Exploration and Exploitation* (Lansing: Michigan State University Press, 2013).
4 Weaver defined a "god term" as "that expression about which all other expressions are ranked as subordinate and serving dominations of power. Its force imparts to others their lesser degree of force and fixes the scale by which degrees of comparison are understood." Richard Weaver, *The Ethics of Rhetoric* (Chicago: H. Regnery Co., 1953), 212.
5 "Smithsonian Explores Beginnings of Biotechnology," *Newsdesk: Newsroom of the Smithsonian*, October 24, 2013, http://newsdesk.si.edu.

6 Donna Haraway, "A Cyborg Manifesto: Science, Technology, and Socialist-Feminism in the Late Twentieth Century," *Simians, Cyborgs, and Women: The Reinvention of Nature* (New York: Routledge, 1991), 150.
7 Kathleen Woodward, "From Virtual Cyborgs to Biological Time Bombs: Technocriticism and the Material Body," in *Culture on the Brink: Ideologies of Technology* (Seattle, WA: Bay Press, 1994): 55.
8 She notes that the cyborg's hybrid standpoint concerns itself with "transgressed boundaries, potent fusions, and dangerous possibilities which progressive people might explore as one part of needed political work." Haraway, "Cyborg Manifesto," 154.
9 Haraway's essay was conceived in a particular historical moment whose contours differ substantially from the time this chapter was written. Haraway has offered detailed accounts of the political transformations that energized the manifesto at the dawn of the Reagan era, especially the complicated, tense, and dismissive positions some feminists adopted toward technology. See, for example, Constance Penley and Andrew Ross, "Cyborgs at Large: Interview with Donna Haraway," *Social Text* 25/26 (1990): 8–23; Nicholas Gane, "When We Have Never Been Human, What Is to Be Done?," *Theory, Culture, Society* 23 (2006): 135–158; Nina Lykke, Randi Markussen, and Finn Olesen, "Cyborgs, Coyotes, and Dogs: A Kinship of Feminist Figurations" and "There are Always More Things Going on than You Thought! Methodologies as Thinking Technologies," *The Haraway Reader* (New York: Routledge, 2004), 321–342.
10 This is not to say that the cyborg is a transhistorical or ahistorical figure. In at least one interview Haraway has insisted it is not. This has not prevented scholars such as Nikolas Rose from making gestures toward this idea. Rose notes, "But were we ever just 'human'—were our capacities ever so natural? I doubt it: humans have never been 'natural' and, at least since the invention of language we have been augmenting our capacities through intellectual, material, and human technologies." For Haraway's explanation, see Gane, "When We Have Never Been Human," 146–147; Nikolas Rose, *The Politics of Life Itself: Biomedicine, Power, and Subjectivity in the Twenty-First Century* (Princeton, NJ: Princeton University Press, 2007), 80.
11 Kenneth Burke, *On Symbols and Society*, ed. Joseph R. Gusfield (Chicago: University of Chicago Press, 1989), 67.
12 Thomas Foster, "Meat Puppets or Robopaths? Cyberpunk and the Question of Embodiment," *Genders* 18 (1993): 14.
13 See Jasbir Puar, "I Would Rather Be a Cyborg Than a Goddess: Becoming-Intersectional in Assemblage Theory," *philoSOPHIA* 2 (2012): 49–66.
14 Haraway's understanding of the cyborg resists origin stories, but that has not stopped her from thinking about the emergence of the concept. She sometimes places the fomentation of this idea in the late nineteenth century, at other times the 1930s, and still other times following the Second World War. What remains unchanged is the conviction that the cyborg is motivated by the relationship

between biologics and informatics on the human body in particular contexts. Humans, she notes, are "products of situated relationalities with organisms, tools, much else." See Gane, "When We Have Never Been Human," 146.
15 Haraway, "Cyborg Manifesto," 152.
16 Idealism and materialism have convoluted histories, often with sudden turns in meaning and contrasting public valences. The two are deeply intertwined in their evolution, representing both a philosophical opposition and more commonly understood distinction between altruism and selfishness. Raymond Williams tells us that idealism, with its complicated intellectual histories, tends to suggest that ideas underline, if not outright constitute, all forms of reality and are fundamental to human consciousness. Williams traces how the term "idealism" eventually morphed into present-day understandings of something that is imaginatively positive or negative (i.e., naïve idealism) and juxtaposes it to other philosophical schools of thought such as materialism and realism. Materialism itself is described as overwhelmingly broad in its scope and aims. Its etymological development is swift and dizzying in Williams's account. He details it as a set of perspectives that are concerned with everything from matter being the "primary substance of all living and non-living things," to a "distinguishable set of attitudes and activities, with no necessary philosophical and scientific connection" that is preoccupied with the "preoccupation or acquisition of things and money." Materialism is connected to the idea of "matter," which was seen as distinct from but necessary to the emergence of form. The notion of materialism was also often contrasted with spiritualism (or ideas) and in many contexts, form and spirit were interconnected. See Raymond Williams, *Keywords: A Vocabulary of Culture and Society* (New York: Oxford University Press, 1976/1983), 152/197.
17 Materialism and idealism make frequent appearances together in humanist scholarship, especially in the mid-twentieth century, and receive special attention in the writings of Kenneth Burke. In *A Grammar of Motives*, Burke contemplates a theory of drama for detailing human motives. The drama metaphor underscores the ongoing tale of humanity and Burke outlines five recurring figures for contemplating human motives: agent, scene, agency, act, and purpose. Burke assigned agent and scene the corresponding philosophies of idealism and materialism, which help to inform the ideas being explored in this chapter. See Kenneth Burke, *A Grammar of Motives* (Berkeley: University of California Press, 1945/1962), 131/171.
18 This analysis resonates strongly with Martha Solomon Watson's writings about the Tuskegee medical experiments and the dehumanization of African American men. See "The Rhetoric of Dehumanization: An Analysis of Medical Reports of the Tuskegee Syphilis Project," *Western Journal of Speech Communication* 49 (1985): 233–247.
19 Although words such as unease, anxiety, and risk tend to preoccupy writings about diabetes history, scientific management, and the cyborg manifesto, Haraway seems to eschew such a language. Indeed, the idea of risk appears only with

regard to the necessity of risky political endeavors and the struggle over meaning-making practices.
20 Haraway, "Cyborg Manifesto," 176.
21 Haraway, "Cyborg Manifesto," 175.
22 Gane, "When We Have Never Been Human," 152. Haraway raises her fascination with tropes (her favorite is metaplasm) in multiple publications. See also "Introduction: A Kinship of Feminist Figurations" and "Morphing in the Order: Flexible Strategies, Feminist Science Studies, and Primate Revisions," both in *The Haraway Reader,* 200–201.
23 Haraway, "Cyborg Manifesto," 163.
24 Gane, "When We Have Never Been Human," 139.
25 Lykke, Markussen, and Olesen, "Cyborgs, Coyotes, and Dogs," 327.
26 Michael Bliss, *The Discovery of Insulin* (Chicago: University of Chicago Press, 1982/2007), 11; Robert Tattersall, *Diabetes: The Biography* (Oxford: Oxford University Press, 2009), 63.
27 See Jenell Johnson, *American Lobotomy: A Rhetorical History* (Ann Arbor: University of Michigan Press, 2014).
28 Chris Feudtner, *Bittersweet: Diabetes, Insulin, and the Transformation of Illness* (Chapel Hill: University of North Carolina Press, 2003), 9.
29 Feudtner, *Bittersweet,* 9.
30 See Plato, *The Phaedrus,* translated by Alexander Nehamas and Paul Woodruff (Indianapolis, IN: Hackett, 1995).
31 Edward Tenner, *Why Things Bite Back: Technology and the Revenge of Unintended Consequences* (New York: Vintage Books, 1997).
32 Feudtner, *Bittersweet,* 68.
33 Feudtner, *Bittersweet,* 100–101.
34 Feudtner, *Bittersweet,* 203.
35 Bliss, *Discovery of Insulin,* 245.
36 Feudtner, *Bittersweet,* 68, 77, 86.
37 Riva Greenberg, "Diabetes' JDRF Tries Shock Ad to Push the FDA," *Huffington Post,* January 16, 2012, http://www.huffingtonpost.com.
38 The word "human" is sometimes put in quotation marks to draw attention to the fact that the insulin is derived from bacteria or yeast.
39 Lawrence Altman, "A New Insulin Given Approval for Use in U.S.," *New York Times,* October 30, 1982.
40 Philip J. Hilts, "Genetic Engineering Starts to Pay," *Washington Post,* December 5, 1982, C5.
41 Daniel Cuff, "Drug Is Expected to Give Lilly Better Image, If Not Profit Rise," *New York Times,* October 30, 1982, 16.
42 Eli Lilly made more than a million dollars from the sale of insulin in the first year it was marketed in the early 1920s. Bliss, *Discovery of Insulin,* 240. In today's market that would be roughly $14 million. We should keep in mind that there were far fewer people with diabetes then than there are today.

43 For more on the concept of "technobiopower," see Gane, "When We Have Never Been Human," 148–149; Federica Timeto, *Diffractive Technospaces: A Feminist Approach to the Mediations of Space and Representation* (Farnham, UK: Ashgate, 2015), 121–122; Sylvia Pritsch, "Inventing Images, Constructing Standpoints: Feminist Strategies of the Technology of the Self," in *Feminism and the Final Foucault*, ed. Diana Taylor and Karen Vintges (Urbana: University of Illinois Press, 2004), 137–138.

44 Robert Metz, "Market Place: Genentech's Outlook Now," *New York Times*, November 1, 1982, D5.

45 Paul Brown, "Diabetics Not Told of Insulin Risk," *The Guardian*, March 8, 1999.

46 Erika Gebel, "Making Insulin: A Behind the Scenes Look at Producing a Lifesaving Medication," *Diabetes Forecast*, July 2013, http://www.diabetesforecast.org; Allan Bruckheim, "Human Insulin May Be Better Than Animal," *Chicago Tribune*, July 29, 1990, http://articles.chicagotribune.com.

47 For the latter, see Carole Blair and Neil Michael, "Commemorating the Theme Park Zone: Reading the Astronauts Memorial," in *At the Intersection: Cultural Studies and Rhetorical Studies*, ed. Thomas Rosteck (New York: Guilford Press, 1998), 29–83.

48 People with diabetes who are not on a pump often require two forms of insulin: a long-lasting form to provide a base (or basal level) and a fast-acting form of insulin when they eat. Pumps eliminate the need for the basal injections, relying exclusively on fast-acting insulin.

49 They cite studies that find a 54 percent reduction in kidney damage, a 41 percent reduction in cardiovascular and nerve damage, and a 53 percent reduction in eye damage. See Medtronic's website at http://www.medtronicdiabetes.com.

50 David Spero, "Is Continuous Glucose Monitoring Worth It?," *Diabetes Self-Management*, September 28, 2011, http://www.diabetesselfmanagement.com.

51 Jonathan D. Rockoff, "J&J Warns Insulin Pump Vulnerable to Cyber Hacking," *Wall Street Journal*, October 4, 2016, http://www.wsj.com.

52 Kathryn Doyle, "Experts Call for Transparency on Insulin Pump Problems," *Reuters*, March 16, 2015, http://www.reuters.com.

53 Doyle, "Experts Call for Transparency."

54 Medtronic touted that the FDA provided an "earlier-than-anticipated approval" for the technology. The same rhetoric was used when the FDA speedily approved "human" insulin decades earlier. Such sentiments clearly contradict the lobbying efforts of the JDRF (discussed in chapter 3) that argued tirelessly that the FDA was erecting unnecessary road blocks to approving such devices.

55 Tim Blotz, "'Game Changer' Device for Type 1 Diabetes Patient Mimics Pancreas," *Fox9.com*, September 15, 2016, http://www.fox9.com/.

56 The night time readings were perhaps more impressive. The study found at night people stayed in range 76.4 percent of the time versus 67.8 percent without the system.

57 JDRF, "JDRF Celebrates Historic Artificial Pancreas Success Bringing Life-changing Benefits to People with Type 1 Diabetes," September 28, 2016, https://www2.jdrf.org.
58 "Introducing Our Smart Contact Lens Project," Google's official blog, January 16, 2014, http://googleblog.blogspot.com.
59 Rachel Barclay, "Google Scientists Create Contact Lens to Measure Blood Sugar Levels in Tears," *Healthline News*, January 23, 2014, http://www.healthline.com.
60 Leo King, "Google Reveals Gigantic Ambitions to Fight Cancer, Diabetes, Parkinson's, Heart Problems," *Forbes*, August 24, 2015, http://www.forbes.com.
61 Kavita Toor, "Google Joins Dexcom to Create Small and Affordable Diabetes Device," *Nature World Report*, August 15, 2015, http://www.natureworldreport.com.
62 Andrew Schneider, "Insulin Price Scandal Hurts Many More Than EpiPen Issues Do," *Montana Standard*, September 4, 2016, http://mtstandard.com.
63 Ben Popken, "Is Insulin the New EpiPen? Families Facing Sticker Shock Over 400 Percent Price Hike," *NBC News*, November 2, 2016, http://www.nbcnews.com.
64 Penley and Ross, "Cyborgs at Large," 18.
65 Alan Jude Ryland, "The EpiPen Wasn't Alone: Price Gouging on Insulin Draws Outrage," *Second Nexus*, September 16, 2016, http://secondnexus.com.
66 Popken, "Is Insulin the New EpiPen?"
67 Ryland, "The EpiPen Wasn't Alone."
68 Caitlin Huston, "Eli Lilly's Revenue Boosted by Jacking Up Cost of Insulin for Diabetics," *Market Watch*, January 29, 2016, http://www.marketwatch.com.
69 Kasia Lipska, "Break Up the Insulin Racket," *New York Times*, February 20, 2016, http://www.nytimes.com.
70 Jeremy A. Green and Kevin Riggs, "Why Is There No Generic Insulin? Historical Origins of a Modern Problem," *New England Journal of Medicine* 372 (2015): 1173.
71 Lipska, "Break Up the Insulin Racket."
72 This is to say nothing of pharmacy benefit managers (PBMs) who negotiate the price of insulin on behalf of insurers. The *New York Times* recently pointed out that PBMs manage a $200 billion industry annually but rarely pass along savings to consumers. See Lipska, "Break Up the Insulin Racket."
73 Green and Riggs, "Why Is There No Generic Insulin?," 1174.
74 Just as the word "human" is a misnomer in "human" insulin, the word "generic" does not quite capture the spirit of the drugs that would be produced. Because insulin is a biologic, it is more complicated to manufacturer than cold medicine or pain relievers. Generic biologics are technically classified as "biosimiliars," which are riskier to make and sometimes have different reactions in the body.

INDEX

A1C: as health indicator, 122, 146, 147, 150, 154, 160; and insurance companies, 160; and marginalized populations, 167, 168; and prevalence reports, 155–156; and privacy, 162; and public health, 40, 142–143, 147, 154, 158, 165; and technology, 107, 191; and Sonia Sotomayor, 113, 122
abstinence, 67–70
ACT-UP, 46, 48
"A Day with HIV in America," 42
Advocate, 56
affinity politics, 195
Affordable Care Act (ACA), 4, 86, 200; access to care, 21, 197; individual mandate, 122; and pre-existing conditions, 160; single payer health insurance, 200
agency, 15–16; and ableism, 125; and Alzheimer's, 75; and apocalyptic discourse, 48; and children, 81; and HIV, 54; lateral agency, 43; patient agency, 15–18, 19, 87, 143; and precarity, 52; and structure, 17, 19, 144; and sovereignty, 8; subjectivity, 15, 22, 191, 197, 200, 201; and technology, 191, 194
AIDS, 25, 137, 156; and abstinence, 67–68; and activism, 47–48, 60, 168; and apocalypse, 47–48; analogies to diabetes, 60–76, 137; and Congressional testimony, 89; and conspiracy theories, 50; and disability, 47, 55; as discursively unstable, 43–48; and metaphors, 74; and paranoia, 50–51; and precarity, 51–52; and public health, 156, 167; and race, 70–71; and retroviral therapy, 49; and shame, 63–64; and vernacular rhetoric, 10–11. *See also* HIV
AIDS Healthcare Foundation, 68
AIDS Memorial Quilt, 48
Akaka, Daniel, 90
Alberti, Danielle, 92
Alcoff, Linda Martín, 113
allegories, 9, 30
Allen, Ray, 80, 110
Alzheimer's disease: registries for, 147; and stem cell research, 77; as "type 3 diabetes," 14, 74–75
American Diabetes Association (ADA), 14, 168, 184, 216n82, 229n25; and activism, 200; differences with JDRF, 78–79; and discrimination, 157
Americans with Disabilities Act (ADA), 29, 55, 114, 130
analogy: between communicable and noncommunicable diseases, 161–162; between HIV and diabetes, 38–39, 42–76, 137; in production of medical knowledge, 42–43; as rhetorical figures, 44
Andriote, Manuel, 58–59, 66
anecdotes: as constitutive, 9; as knowledge, 27, 30; and JDRF, 98; and prudence, 131; and Sonia Sotomayor, 131, 134–135, 136
Angels in America, 48
Anzaldúa, Gloria, 1, 23–24, 36; and type 1 diabetes, 118–119

239

apocalypse, 39, 45, 48, 201; and agency, 48–49; and AIDS, 47–48; and art, 48; and global diabetes rates, 75; and group politics, 49; as "secular" or "civil," 49; as trope, 48; and utopia, 48, 49, 51, 52
artificial pancreas, 30, 86, 110; and JDRF, 99–100, 104–108, 189, 200; and medical frontier, 41, 176–177, 189, 192–194; and patient reception, 192–194
Auchincloss, Hugh, 101–102

Ball, Howard, 121
Bayer, Ronald, 157
Begich, Mark, 106–108
Bennett, Robert, 88
Bennett, Tony, 80
Berlant, Lauren, 27, 37, 59; diva citizenship, 83; infantile citizenship, 83; and lateral agency, 43; and slow death, 53
Berry, Cleo, 171
Berry, Halle, 29
Beyond Type 1 (blog), 200
biosimilars (generic insulin), 41, 185, 199
Birth of Biotech exhibit, 173–177, 186
Bliss, Michael, 183
Bloomberg, Michael, 168
Bonness, Eric, 96
boyd, danah, 82
breast cancer, 21, 161, 207n10, 201n48
Brimley, Wilfred, 29
British Diabetes Association, 186
Bronx, 40, 113, 141, 147, 168
Brown, Scott, 106
Bryant, Anita, 81
Burke, Kenneth, 73, 178, 228n12, 229n29, 234n17
Bush, George, 77–78, 85, 86, 101–104, 128
Butler, Judith, 51–52

capitalism, 27; and insulin, 173, 195, 196–201; and precarity, 53
Carnahan, Jean, 87

Center for Disease Control (CDC), 144
Chamany, Shadi, 151, 155–156, 162, 163, 166
Chávez, Karma, 117
childhood (as modern invention), 81
children: and access to medicine, 200; and advocacy, 77–111; and civic identity, 81, 83; as cultural contradiction, 82; and discovery of insulin, 82; and history of diabetes, 83, 173–175, 183, 186; and Humulin, 186; and management discourses, 84; and normality, 92, 93–94; as symbol of nationalism, 81, 100; and type 1 diabetes, 11, 20, 64
Children's Congress, as a study in form, 89. *See also* JDRF
chronic conditions: and agency, 19–22; and depression, 4, 66–67; development of diabetes as, 83–84; as ephemeral, 115; history of, 15–16, 75; HIV as, 39, 43–46, 49, 61–63; and precarity, 51; and public health, 142–172; relationship to time, 34, 56, 59, 177; and technology, 179
cicadas (as symbol of restraint), 1–2
Cisneros, Josue David, 114
civic humanism, 143
Clinton, Bill, 121
Clinton, Hillary, 88
Coates, Ta-Nehisi, 120
Cohen, Cathy, 71
Colburn, Tom, 128
Colgrove, James, 157
Collins, Susan, 86, 88, 90, 96, 101, 106
Comenius, Johan Amos, 81
coming out, 26
condensation symbols, 7, 8, 184, 207n9
Conrad, Peter, 17, 21, 22
continuous glucose monitors (CGMs), 86, 159; and cost, 201; and cyborg sensibilities, 179; in JDRF rhetoric, 105, 107–109; and technological development, 189–195
control: and agency, 18, 201; as abstract goal, 15, 96–97; and civility, 123; and

HIV, 39, 44, 67; and morality, 19, 67–69, 75, 97, 110, 114, 119, 122, 154; as obligation, 13, 160; projections of ease, 8, 62, 91; and prudence, 40, 119; and public health, 144–147, 152–156; and Sonia Sotomayor, 113, 122–129, 132–133; and technology, 188–193
Cornyn, John, 129, 131
costs: of insulin, 185, 188, 196–201; medical, 22, 41, 55, 58, 176, 182; national budgets, 9, 21, 85, 110; New York City, 147, 159–160; and prevention programs, 21; and technology, 107, 184–185, 193
Craig, Larry, 86
cripistemologies, 116–117
CrossFit, 68–69
Cutler, Jay, 29
Cvetkovich, Ann, 47, 67
cyborg, 41, 178–181, 189, 194, 195, 201; and artificial pancreas, 100, 104
Cyborg Manifesto, 177–182, 199
Cygnarowicz, Sophia, 94, 98

Davidson, Mayer, 197
dawn phenomenon (also dawn effect), 33
depression, 4, 5, 9, 19, 66–67, 76, 118; analogies to, 43; and war metaphors, 87
diabetes: and allegories, 9, 30; analogies to noncommunicable disease, 161–162; analogies to HIV, 38–39, 42–76, 137; and condensation symbols, 7,8, 184, 207n9; and costs, 9, 21–22, 85, 110; and discrimination, 157; etymology, 3, 46; and film, 11, 28; gestational, 11, 14–15; and life expectancy, 9, 43; and metaphor, 7, 73–74, 138, 177, 180; as national crisis, 9; and race, 11–13, 71–73, 118, 169–172; vernacular interpretations of, 10–11. *See also* type 1 diabetes; type 2 diabetes
diabetes registry programs, 40, 142–172; and prevalence reports, 154–156; and public health, 142, 148–150, 165–168; and privacy, 143, 156–164. *See also* patient registries
diabetic ketoacidosis, 3, 11, 14, 183; and insulin pumps, 190–192, 194
diabulimia, 30
Diagnostic and Statistical Manual of Mental Disorders (DSM), 25
disability, 25, 27, 29, 37; and childhood, 84; and citizenship, 13, 84; and diabetes, 114; and intersectionality, 114–117, 138; and productivity, 19; and queer theory, 47; and race, 13, 40, 171; as resisting normality, 92; and Sonia Sotomayor, 125, 129, 131, 136, 139–141
disability critical race theory (DisCrit), 116
diva citizenship, 83
Donnelly, William, 16
Dow, Bonnie, 54
Dudley, Rachel, 95
Duggan, Lisa, 115
Durbin, Dick, 127
Duster, Troy, 72, 118

Eisenhower, Dwight, 121
Elias, Norbert, 208n22
Eli Lilly, 185–187, 197–198, 235n42
epidemics, 7, 10, 23, 40; etymology, 151; Foucault on, 145; as inciting urgency, 144, 150, 152, 170; as metaphor, 145, 148–149, 167, 172, 202; as public health descriptor, 151–152, 170; as resource generator, 150, 162, 202; scrutinized 145, 161–162, 168–171; and surveillance, 155
evergreening, 41, 198–200

Fairchild, Amy, 157
fatalism, 5, 23, 38, 146, 184–185, 197, 201–202, 207n3; and JDRF, 39, 76, 79–80, 84, 91, 99, 103, 109, 186; and technology, 191, 194

Feinstein, Diane, 129
feminist politics, 25, 37, 179, 195
Ferzacca, Steve, 17
Feudtner, Chris, 83, 182–183
Field, Sally, 28
Flores, Lisa, 114
Food and Drug Administration (FDA), 105–107, 179, 186, 192, 213n21
Foster, Tom, 178
Foucault, Michel, 16, 17, 27, 54, 60; and clinical health, 145; and statistics, 98
Franken, Al, 129
Frieden, Thomas, 144
Frist, Bill, 78

Genentech, 173, 181
gestational diabetes, 11, 14
Getty, Jeff, 55
Gilman, Sander, 153
Ginsburg, Ruth Bader, 121, 140
Goldman, Janlori, 157, 158, 163
Goldstein, Tom, 128
Google, 195
Gould, Ellen, 90, 91
Gould, Patrick, 109
Graham, Lindsey, 128, 130
Graham, S. Scott, 61
Grassley, Chuck, 129
Green, Jeremy, 185, 199
Griffin, Cindy, 117

Hahner, Leslie, 117–118
Halasz, Katie, 97
Hall, Gary, 80
Hanson, Ellis, 47
Happe, Kelly, 72
Haraway, Donna, 41, 177–182, 195, 199, 202; and tropes, 180–181
Harper, Phillip Brian, 71
Hawkins, Tré, 94
health (as social construct), 6, 43
Hering, Bernhard, 102–103

HIV: and abstinence, 67–68; analogies to diabetes, 38, 42–76, 137, 162; as a chronic condition, 16, 39, 45–46; as discursively unstable 43, 45, 55; and disease registries, 146, 157; and metaphor, 60; and paranoia, 50–51, 56, 58–59; and precarity, 51–52; and queer theory, 25, 45; and race, 70–72; and shame, 63–64; and vernacular rhetorics, 10–11
Hoppin, Margaret, 158, 159, 161–162
How to Have Theory in an Epidemic, 10
Humulin, 184–187, 199
hyperglycemia, 11, 14, 34, 190
hypoglycemia, 11, 18, 28, 29, 30, 34, 36, 97, 114; and discovery of insulin, 83; and new insulins, 184, 186; and stem cell treatment, 102–103

idealism, 179, 234n16
infantile citizenship, 83, 168
infectious disease, 15, 21; analogies to diabetes, 142, 144, 151, 154, 161–162; and HIV, 16
"inspiration porn," 84, 116
insulin: and Alzheimer's, 14, 74; animal-based, 175, 184, 188; and biosimilars (generics), 41, 185, 198–200; and capitalism, 173, 184–185, 196–200; and children, 82; discovery of, 46, 82–83, 99, 175, 182–185; function of, 11–12; and history, 173; and hypoglycemia, 11, 18; and islet transplants, 102–103; and prudence, 138; and recombinant DNA, 173–176; synthetic, 175–177; and technology ethos, 182
Insulin for Life USA, 200
insulin pump, 7, 11, 179, 181, 189–194; and artificial pancreas, 105, 107
International Diabetes Federation, 200
intersectionality: and critique, 116–118, 129; as rhetorical form, 117
islet cells, 54, 101–103

Jack, Belinda, 24
Jacobs, Jen, 30–37
JDRF, 76–111, 168, 183; and artificial pancreas, 104–108, 192, 200; and diva citizenship, 83; and fatalism, 39, 76, 146, 186, 201; fundraising, 79, 85; lobbying White House, 78; and normality, 92–94; and science, 99–108; and Special Diabetes Program (SDP), 85; and stem cells, 100–104; transcending partisanship, 88; and type 2 diabetes, 110–111; and use of statistical data, 98
Johnson, Jenell, 182
Jonas, Nick, 29, 69, 80, 90
Jones, Aaron, 93
judgment: and condensation symbols, 207n9; and emotion, 135; and prudence, 20, 48, 119; and relationship to management, 8, 114–115; surveillance, 35, 148

Kelly, Asa, 93
Keränen, Lisa, 150
Kern, Rochelle, 21
Klein, Kevin, 80
Kleinman, Arthur, 16
Kramer, Larry, 48
Krent, Harold, 158, 159, 160
Kuppers, Petra, 211–212n68
Kushner, Tony, 48
Kyl, Jon, 128

Latent Autoimmune Diabetes in Adults (LADA), 13
Lautenberg, Frank, 86–87
Law, John, 18
Lazarus effect, 100, 103, 196
Leahy, Patrick, 129
LeBesco, Kathleen, 70
Leonard, Sugar Ray, 80
Levin, Carl, 87
liberalism, 143, 159, 160
life expectancy rates (for people with diabetes), 9, 43

Long, Thomas, 48
Lorde, Audre, 24
Love, Heather, 213n26
Lovell, James, 80, 90
Lynch, John, 101
Lyon, Roger Gail, 89

Majdik, Zoltan, 16
management: and agency, 15–19; and allegories, 9, 30; and analogy, 59, 63, 66; case studies, 38–41; and choice, 59–60; and community action, 75, 143–146; as condensation symbol, 8–9; as contested concept, 7; focus on the clinic, 8, 17, 23; history of chronic conditions, 15–16; and the humanities, 23–24, 38; internal contradictions of, 18; and judgment, 8, 114–115; and medicalization, 17; as personal transcendence, 116; and productivity, 19; and prudence, 20, 48, 119; and race, 12, 70; as rhetorical construct, 20–21, 25; and tropes, 7, 38, 44–45, 64, 180–181, 186; vernacular interpretations of, 10, 26–27
Mariner, Wendy, 158, 160, 161
Martin, Emily, 23
materialism, 179, 234n16
Mature Onset Diabetes of the Young (MODY), 14
McEnery, Caroline, 90, 94, 107–108
McKinnon, Sara, 117
McTigue, Kathleen, 151
medicalization, 17
Medtronic, 106, 189–193, 200
metaphor: bodies as machines, 179; and diabetes, 7, 73–74, 138, 177, 180; and epidemics, 144–145, 148, 161, 167, 202; food deserts, 72; and HIV/AIDS, 60, 70, 73–74; and insulin, 196; legal, 159; and obesity, 153; war, 87, 91–92, 149. *See also* trope

Michaels, Bret, 29
Mitchell, Gordon, 151
Mol, Annemarie, 5, 17, 18, 19, 37
Moore, Mary Tyler, 29, 80, 90–93, 103
Morgan, Kerry, 90
Morris, Charles E., 82, 139
Morris, David, 18
Morris, Stockton, 94
Morrison, Adam, 80, 90
Muñoz, José Esteban, 113, 130, 139
Murray, Patty, 87
My Beloved World (Sotomayor), 115, 133–138

narrative: and AIDS, 43, 45; American Dream, 40, 113; as constitutive, 9, 149; personal narrative, 27, 37, 88, 108, 133–138, 140; and personal responsibility, 4; and restraint, 6, 13, 30, 112, 116; and science, 102
national identity, 84, 173
National Institute of Health (NIH), 85, 88, 90, 101, 102
National Institute of Mental Health (NIMH), 19
nationalism, 10, 71, 81–82, 100, 114
National Museum of American History (Smithsonian), 173–177, 186
Nelson, Ben, 109–110
New York City: cost of diabetes to city, 147; hospital system, 166; populations affected by diabetes, 147; rates of diabetes, 146
New York City Department of Health and Mental Hygiene (DOHMH), 30, 40, 142–172
Nip/Tuck, 53
noncommunicable diseases, 144, 166
normality, 83, 88, 92, 93–94, 98–99
Novo Nordisk, 197

Obama, Barack, 40, 67, 112–113, 121, 123, 126, 136, 139, 144

Obama, Michelle, 153
obesity, 24, 74, 150–151, 155; as epidemic, 152–153, 161, 169–171
O'Connor, Sandra Day, 112, 121, 140

The Panic Room, 11
paranoid readings: and diabetes, 75, 62; and form, 50, 56; and HIV/AIDS, 45, 47, 49–51, 54, 56, 59; and JDRF, 84; and queer studies, 50–51; and reparative readings 50–51, 52; and shame, 64; and technology, 181
patient registries, 142, 164; and personal data, 158; Vermont registry, 229n25. *See also* diabetes registry programs
Patriot Act, 161
Patton, Cindy, 152, 155
Pemberton, Max, 62
Perelman, Chaïm, 44, 69
personal responsibility, 4, 14, 69, 165, 194; and liberalism, 143; and race, 70–71; and technology, 192
Pezzullo, Phaedra, 207n10
Plato (*Phaedrus*), 1–2, 23–24, 182–183
Platt, Carrie Ann, 16
Poe, Bob, 61
precarity, 39, 45, 47, 74, 75, 122; defined, 51; and HIV/AIDS, 51–52
pre-existing conditions, 160, 201
pre-exposure prophylaxis (PrEP), 51, 57, 68, 69
prevalence reports, 145, 147, 155–56, 162, 229n25
privacy: and diabetes registry programs, 40, 143–146, 156–163, 165, 167–168; and diabetes technology, 190–191
productivity (social models of), 19, 114
prudence, 20, 105, 115, 191; and Sonia Sotomayor, 40, 113–115, 119, 123, 126, 139
Pryor, Mark, 107
public health: and discourse, 149; and epidemics, 144–146, 148–153, 161–162; and HIV/AIDS, 46–47, 62, 67–68; and

management, 16–17; New York City, 30, 142–172; and noncommunicable disease, 142–143; and privacy, 156–164; and Sonia Sotomayor, 130, 141; and surveillance, 146

queer theory: and apocalypse, 48–49; and children, 81–82, 84; and criticism, 25–29, 37; and HIV/AIDS, 45, 47–48, 50, 52, 137; and paranoid readings, 48–51; and precarity, 51–53
Queerty, 42, 44

race: analogies between diabetes and HIV, 10, 39, 70–73; and disability, 40, 116; and genetics, 72; and intersectionality, 115–119, 129, 130, 138, 139; and media reports, 12–13; and public health campaigns, 169–172; and typologies of diabetes, 12–13, 72, 118
Rand, Erin, 215n61
Reagan, Nancy, 78, 104
Reagan, Ronald, 63, 233n9
recombinant DNA, 173–176, 179, 184
reparative readings: and form, 62; and JDRF, 84; and paranoid readings, 50–51; and public health, 146; and "weak theories," 51
revenge effects, 83, 183
Rhodes, Dennis, 55, 59
Riggs, Kevin, 185, 199
Roberts, John, 121–122, 130, 140
Roberts, Julia, 28–29
Rose, Nikolas, 233n10
Rosen, Jeffrey, 119–121, 132–133
Rowley, Caroline, 77, 96

Sanofi, 197
Savage, Dan, 81
scapegoating, 6, 67, 73, 157
Schumer, Chuck, 132
Scott, Laniece Evans, 95, 97

Sedgwick, Eve Kosofsky, 24, 47; on paranoia, 56; on paranoid and reparative readings, 50–51; on the reparative, 62
Segal, Judy, 149
Sessions, Jeff, 112
Shaheen, Jeanne, 87, 106–107
shame, 5, 10, 20, 39, 63–67, 95, 149, 172; in diabetes communities, 26, 64–67, 76, 163, 194; and HIV, 60, 63–64; and restraint, 67–69; and surveillance, 13, 20, 171–172
Shaw, Theodore, 127
Siebers, Tobin, 125
Singer, Mollie, 95, 98
single-payer healthcare, 22, 146, 200
slow death, 7, 53, 79, 100, 199, 201
Smart, Jean, 80
Smith, Will, 94
Smithsonian, 173–177, 186
Snorton, C. Riley, 71
Socrates, 1–2, 23, 36
Solomon, River, 66
Sontag, Susan, 24, 47, 70; and the epidemic frame, 145
Sotomayor, Sonia, 29, 39–40, 111–141; confirmation hearings, 126–133; and control, 122–24; and judicial restraint, 126–133; and media narratives, 119–126, 132; and memoir, 115, 133–138; *My Beloved World*, 115, 133–138; and personal transcendence, 113, 116, 127; and prudence, 114–115, 124–126; and "wise Latina" speech, 112, 119
Special Diabetes Program (SDP), 85, 108
Spiegel, Allen, 90, 102
Stanford, Lauren, 98
Steel Magnolias, 11, 28–29
Stein, Sam, 122
stem cells, 78, 86, 100–105
stigma, 19, 20, 69, 97, 148, 167, 172; and HIV, 42–43, 47, 53, 58–60, 62–63, 67; and type 2 diabetes, 64, 66, 69, 73–74, 157, 163

Stockton, Kathryn Boyd, 81, 94
Stoics, 208n22
Stolberg, Sheryl Gay, 123
Stone, Mary Specker, 17, 21
Strader, Ann, 90
Strauss, Anselm, 22
"structure of feeling," 23
Sullivan, Andrew, 56–60, 70–71
"super crip," 40, 84, 116
Supreme Court (health of nominees), 121

Taft, William, 121
Tarver, Erin, 140
Taylor, Frederick, 208n22
technobiopower, 185, 236n43
Test Positive Aware Network (TPAN), 42
Thurmond, Strom, 78, 87
Toobin, Jeffrey, 121
Tomes, Nancy, 149–150, 167
Treichler, Paula, 7, 10–11, 47, 60
Trump, Donald, 160, 197
trope: apocalypse as, 48; children as, 80, 173; of choice in management discourse, 60, 177; as constitutive, 148; epidemic as, 145, 152, 165, 168, 171–172; fatalism as, 103, 201; in Haraway's work, 180; management as, 7, 38, 44–45, 64; 180–181, 186; metaphors for diabetes, 74; normality as, 93; paranoia as, 50; of personal responsibility, 71, 114, 159. *See also* metaphor
Tuchman, Arleen Marcia, 216n75
tudiabetes.com, 28
type 1 diabetes: adult onset, 20, 64; in art, 30–37; characteristics of, 11; and children, 82, 174–76, 186–187; conflicts with people with type 2 diabetes, 6, 65–66, 194; confusion about, 10; contrasted to type 2 diabetes, 6, 13, 64; and economic hardship, 21–22; in film, 28–29; and race, 72; and stem cells, 101–102
type 2 diabetes, 10, 11, 12, 20; characteristics of, 11–12; conflicts with people with type 1 diabetes, 65–66, 194; confusion about, 10, 176; contrasted to type 1 diabetes, 13; and JDRF, 110–111; and prescription costs, 198–199; and public health, 148, 170; and race, 11–12, 72, 118; result of HIV medication, 54; and stigma, 6, 14, 64
"type 3 diabetes," 14, 74–75. *See also* Alzheimer's disease

utopia: and abstinence, 68; and apocalypse 48, 51–52

Varmus, Harold, 100

Wald, Pricilla, 145, 149, 151
Walters, Clint, 55, 56, 59
Warner, Michael, 27
Weaver, Richard, 176, 232n4
Webber, Andrew, 97
West, Isaac, 44
Whitehouse, Sheldon, 129, 130
whiteness, 12; and children with type 1 diabetes, 72, 174, 186; and Congress, 126, 128; and genetics, 72; and judicial sphere, 115, 119, 135; and respectability politics, 26–27
Wick, Douglas, 104
Williams, Raymond, 23, 234n16
Woolf, Virginia, 24

Zimliki, Chip, 105–107

ABOUT THE AUTHOR

Jeffrey A. Bennett is Associate Professor of Communication Studies at Vanderbilt University. He is the author of *Banning Queer Blood: Rhetorics of Citizenship, Contagion, and Resistance*. He has lived with type 1 diabetes since 2004.

www.ingramcontent.com/pod-product-compliance
Lightning Source LLC
Chambersburg PA
CBHW020250030426

42336CB00010B/698